Hypertension

YOUR QUESTION

This book is dedicated to the memory of Mrs Joan Cockcroft

Commissioning Editor: Ellen Green
Project Development and Management: Fiona Conn
Design: Jayne Jones, George Ajayi, Keith Kail

Hypertension:

YOUR QUESTIONS ANSWERED

Ian B Wilkinson
BM BCh MA MRCP
Lecturer in Clinical Pharmacology,
The University of Cambridge,
and Honorary Consultant Physician,
Addenbrooke's Hospital NHS Trust,
Cambridge, UK

W Stephen Waring
BMedSci MB BCh BAO MRCP
Lecturer in Clinical Pharmacology
and Specialist Registrar in Medicine,
The University of Edinburgh, UK

John R Cockcroft
BSc (Hons) MB ChB FRCP
Professor, The University of Wales College of Medicine,
and Honorary Consultant in Cardiology,
Wales Heart Research Institute, Cardiff, UK

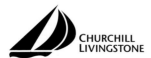

CHURCHILL
LIVINGSTONE

EDINBURGH LONDON NEW YORK PHILADELPHIA ST LOUIS SYDNEY TORONTO 2003

CHURCHILL LIVINGSTONE
An imprint of Elsevier Science Limited

First published 2003

ISBN 0 443 07255 8

British Library Cataloguing in Publication Data
A catalogue record for this book is available from the British Library

Library of Congress Cataloging in Publication Data
A catalog record for this book is available from the Library of Congress

Note
Medical knowledge is constantly changing. As new information becomes available, changes in treatment, procedures, equipment and the use of drugs become necessary. The authors and the publishers have taken care to ensure that the information given in this text is accurate and up to date. However, readers are strongly advised to confirm that the information, especially with regard to drug usage, complies with the latest legislation and standards of practice.

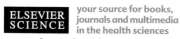

your source for books,
journals and multimedia
in the health sciences
www.elsevierhealth.com

The
publisher's
policy is to use
paper manufactured
from sustainable forests

Typesetting by RDC Tech Group
Printed in China by RDC Group Limited

Contents

Preface

Hypertension is a common disorder affecting about 20% of adults worldwide and over 10 million adults in the UK. Blood pressure rises with age, and thus the prevalence of hypertension increases from about 25% in the middle-aged population, to around 50% in those aged over 75. As a major, but modifiable, risk factor for coronary heart disease, cerebrovascular disease, chronic renal failure and congestive heart failure, it is, therefore, vital that hypertension is both correctly identified and adequately controlled. However, as we enter a new millennium, many patients with raised blood pressure remain undetected and, even when hypertension is diagnosed, a substantial proportion of individuals are under-treated.

Blood pressure was first measured by Stephen Hales in 1711. However, it was not until 1896 that the modern era of blood pressure measurement began, with the introduction of the first syphgmomanometer by Riva-Rocci. Measurements of blood pressure were then rapidly incorporated into basic clinical practice, but there was considerable controversy and debate as to their value in predicting morbidity and mortality. However, by 1920, physicians working for life insurance companies had amassed sufficient data to demonstrate, beyond doubt, that hypertension was a significant risk factor for cardiovascular disease. Nevertheless, controversy as to the pathophysiology of hypertension remained, and there was little in the way of effective therapeutic intervention.

The modern era of antihypertensive therapy began in the 1950s. Thiazide diuretics were introduced into clinical practice in 1959, and the subsequent 50 years saw an explosion of antihypertensive agents targeted at the physiological mechanisms known to maintain normal blood pressure. However, progress has not been without its problems. Despite the plethora of large randomized placebo-controlled, and comparative trials which have already been undertaken, many sponsored by the pharmaceutical industry, it remains unclear as to whether blood pressure reduction per se or the specific class of antihypertensive drug used is of greatest importance in terms of outcome. Indeed, the sheer amount of data generated and the varying quality of the trials has itself added to the confusion amongst clinicians, many of whom are not specifically trained in the management of hypertension but, nevertheless, see many patients with this important condition on a routine basis.

This book is also written at a time which has seen a paradigm shift, away from the pre-eminence of diastolic pressure as the component of blood pressure which best predicts risk, and towards systolic and pulse pressure. It would seem, therefore, that yet again we are on the threshold of another new era in the treatment of blood pressure, in that large numbers of patients now present with isolated systolic hypertension, a disease characterized by large artery stiffness rather than increased peripheral resistance. These individuals represent a renewed challenge in terms of pathophysiology and therapy.

The concept and outline for this book were written by IBW and JRC whilst Visiting Professors at the University of New South Wales in Sydney in 2001. It is intended to guide the clinician interested in hypertension through the potential minefield by concentrating on the most frequently asked and important questions, and by providing, where possible, simple, evidence-based answers. In doing so we also hope to appeal to other health-care professionals interested in hypertension and patients concerned about their own health.

IBW
JRC
WSW

How to use this book

The *Your Questions Answered* series aims to meet the information needs of GPs and other primary care professionals who care for patients with chronic conditions. It is designed to help them work with patients and their families, providing effective, evidence-based care and management.

The books are in an accessible question and answer format, with detailed contents lists at the beginning of every chapter and a complete index to help find specific information.

ICONS

Icons are used in the book to identify particular types of information:

 highlights important information

 highlights side-effect information.

PATIENT QUESTIONS

At the end of relevant chapters there are sections of frequently asked patient questions, with easy-to-understand answers aimed at the non-medical reader. These questions are also listed at the end of the book.

What is hypertension?

1

CLASSIFICATION OF HYPERTENSION

1.1 Can we define hypertension?

It is impossible to provide a precise definition of hypertension since blood pressure is a continuous variable within the population, having a skewed normal distribution. Moreover, cardiovascular risk is continuously related to blood pressure and, therefore, any definition will be purely arbitrary. However, hypertension can be considered as a level of blood pressure that is associated with a significantly increased risk of cardiovascular disease, compared to the population as a whole, and one that is likely to benefit from treatment. From a practical point of view, most authorities would consider a sustained blood pressure of ≥140/90 mmHg as being 'hypertensive' (World Health Organization, WHO – International Society of Hypertension, ISH definition). Nevertheless, a significant proportion of hypertension-related disease occurs in those individuals considered to be 'normotensive', because the majority of the population will have a blood pressure <140/90 mmHg. Therefore, it is important to take into account an individual's overall risk of cardiovascular disease when deciding whether he or she should be labelled as 'hypertensive'.

1.2 How can hypertension be classified?

Hypertension may be classified by aetiology into *essential* or primary hypertension – cause unknown; or *secondary* hypertension where a cause has been identified, e.g. renal artery stenosis. Hypertension may also be divided into '*malignant*' or accelerated-phase and '*benign*' forms, although use of the latter has fallen out of favour since all forms of hypertension carry an increased risk of cardiovascular disease. Categorization can also be based on severity (*Table 1.1*), although again such definitions are purely

TABLE 1.1 Categorization of hypertension by severity (JNC VI)		
Category	Systolic (mmHg)	Diastolic (mmHg)
Normal	< 130	and	< 85
High-normal	130–139	or	85–89
Hypertension			
Stage 1	140–159	or	90–99
Stage 2	160–179	or	100–109
Stage 3	≥ 180	or	≥ 110

Based on the recommendations of the report of the Sixth Joint National Committee (JNC VI) on Prevention, Detection, Evaluation and Treatment of High Blood Pressure (1997).

arbitrary. The term '*resistant hypertension*' is also widely used when hypertension is refractory to 'standard' therapy, e.g. elevated pressures in patients receiving three different antihypertensive drugs.

1.3 What is the most common form of hypertension?

Hypertension affects approximately 1 in 5 of the population overall, but is relatively more common in older age groups. Essential hypertension accounts for between 90 and 95% of all cases, with a variety of secondary causes making up the remainder (*Box 9.1*). However, the exact proportions depend on a number of factors including patient selection, age, and how hard one looks for a cause. Indeed, secondary hypertension is relatively more common amongst younger patients and amongst those with refractory hypertension. Malignant hypertension is now very rare in western societies, although it is also relatively more common in younger individuals and those of African descent.

1.4 Is all essential hypertension the same?

No, essential hypertension is increasingly recognized as a heterogeneous condition, which no doubt reflects the many different contributory factors. Perhaps the most important clinical distinction is between individuals with isolated systolic hypertension and those with elevated diastolic and/or systolic pressures. 'Classical' essential hypertension tends to be associated with the latter form of blood pressure elevation, and is more common in the under-50s. In contrast, isolated systolic hypertension is almost exclusively a disease of older individuals (*Fig. 1.1*). Such observations, together with differing underlying pathophysiological causes, reinforce the notion that they are distinct conditions.

1.5 What is malignant hypertension?

Malignant hypertension, also referred to as accelerated-phase hypertension, is used to describe hypertension associated with retinal haemorrhages or papilloedema. Haemolytic anaemia, renal impairment, proteinuria and haematuria may also be present, and the diastolic blood pressure is often, but not always, >120 mmHg. Malignant hypertension is usually associated with a rapid rise in arterial pressure, and untreated leads to expeditious end-organ damage including cardiac failure and hypertensive encephalopathy. Its pathological hallmark is fibrinoid necrosis of the arterioles and hyperplastic arteriolitis of the arterioles and arteries ('onion skinning'). The incidence of malignant hypertension is about 2 per 100 000 per year, but it is relatively more common in younger adults, males and black people. There is an increased chance of secondary hypertension, and in contrast to those with 'typical' essential hypertension, patients often have symptoms at the time of presentation (*Box 1.1*).

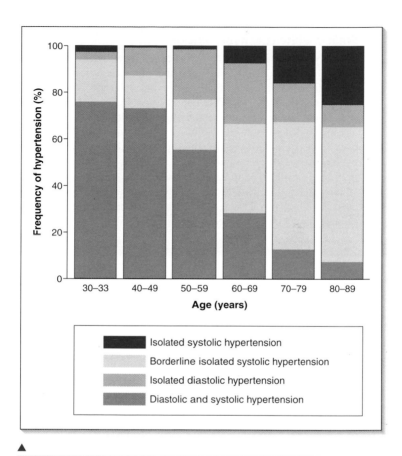

Fig. 1.1 Types of hypertension by age. The frequency of the various categories of hypertension by decade in men. (From Sagie *et al* 1993, with permission. Copyright © 1993 Massachusetts Medical Society. All rights reserved.)

BOX 1.1 Symptoms associated with malignant hypertension

- Blurred vision
- Headache
- Anxiety, confusion, coma
- Seizures
- Chest pain
- Breathlessness
- Nausea, vomiting

1.6 What is white-coat hypertension?

White-coat hypertension refers to the circumstance where an individual's blood pressure is elevated when measured in the clinical situation, e.g. an outpatient clinic, but is 'normal' when assessed outside this setting. This has also been termed 'isolated office hypertension' by some. The true prevalence of the condition is difficult to establish, because various techniques for assessing blood pressure and definitions for 'normal' blood pressure have been applied, but it may be present in up to 15% of subjects with clinical hypertension. However, up to 75% of individuals with white-coat hypertension will go on to develop sustained hypertension within 5 years (Bidlingmeyer *et al* 1996). Moreover, some studies (Strandberg & Salomaa 2000), although not all, suggest that white-coat hypertension is itself associated with increased cardiovascular risk.

EPIDEMIOLOGY

1.7 What is the distribution of blood pressure in the population?

Blood pressure has a skewed normal distribution, and is associated with a continuous spectrum of risk across populations. This unimodal pattern of blood pressure distribution indicates that hypertension is a polygenic disorder, arising as a result of several environmental or genetic influences. Furthermore, this pattern of blood pressure distribution is consistent with the theory that interventions which reduce blood pressure across a population, even by a small degree, could substantially reduce the prevalence of hypertension.

1.8 What is the incidence and prevalence of hypertension in the UK population?

The prevalence of hypertension increases significantly with age, consistent with the age-related rise in blood pressure observed in most populations (*Fig. 1.2*). Indeed, the Health Survey for England reported the prevalence of hypertension to be 3.3% in those aged < 40 years; 27.9% in those aged 40–79 years; and 49.9% in those aged 80 years and over. In the North of England Study, hypertension was identified in 50.3% of primary care patients aged 65–80 years, in whom only 30.0% had achieved adequate blood pressure control (< 150/90 mmHg) and only 13.5% had attained optimal blood pressure control (< 140/85 mmHg). These data suggest that the prevalence of hypertension is between 30 and 50% in the over-65s, but that in practice a significantly lower proportion of patients are actually identified, treated and ultimately attain good blood pressure control.

Certain studies indicate that the incidence of systolic and diastolic hypertension is falling, particularly among young adults, possibly as a result

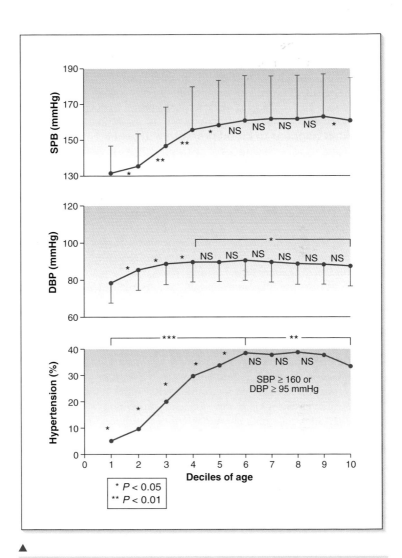

Fig. 1.2 Age and hypertension. Trends in systolic blood pressure (SBP), diastolic blood pressure (DBP), and prevalence of hypertension (SBP ≥160 or DBP ≥95 mmHg) across deciles of age. (From Casiglia & Palatini 1998, with permission of the Nature Publishing Group.)

of health-orientated lifestyle and dietary changes. However, this effect is substantially overwhelmed by the burden imposed by growing numbers of elderly patients in western societies, and the increasing incidence of type 2 diabetes mellitus, with which hypertension often coexists. Therefore, the prevalence of hypertension and cardiovascular disease is rising, and it poses an even greater potential threat to public health in the future.

1.9 What happens to blood pressure with age?

In almost all societies blood pressure rises with advancing age, and until recently this was accepted as an inevitable and benign part of the 'ageing process'. However, although systolic pressure rises progressively throughout life, diastolic blood pressure rises modestly until the age of 50 years and then falls; thus pulse pressure (systolic − diastolic pressure) actually increases after middle-age (*Fig. 1.3*). Importantly, we now recognize that such widening of pulse pressure is associated with a significant increase in cardiovascular morbidity and mortality and, therefore, can no longer be considered as either physiologically 'normal' or benign. Indeed, pulse pressure increases because of progressive arterial stiffening (arteriosclerosis) − a process that appears to be accelerated in certain individuals, and in those with established cardiovascular risk factors such as diabetes mellitus.

1.10 Does blood pressure rise with age in all populations and races?

Although blood pressure rises with age in almost all modern populations, this seems to reflect continued exposure to a number of environmental factors, which results in progressive arterial stiffening, rather than any intrinsic physiological process. Evidence supporting this view comes from observations of certain non-urbanized communities in whom ageing is not associated with rising blood pressure. For example, the Kuna are island dwellers in the Panamanian Caribbean in whom blood pressure does not rise throughout life, and in whom hypertension is very uncommon. Additionally, in those who migrate to the urbanized Panama City, the prevalence of hypertension increases to 10.7%, and exceeds 45% in those over 60 years of age, indicating that age-related blood pressure patterns depend on exposure to other environmental factors.

1.11 Is birth weight related to blood pressure?

The link between low birth weight and later development of high blood pressure was identified over a decade ago, and has been established by various epidemiological reports – the 'Barker' hypothesis (Law *et al* 1993). The mechanisms underlying the association are not clear but may reflect the influence of nutritional factors during gestation; this is supported, in part, by the observation that the extent of nutritional support given to preterm infants can also determine adult blood pressure. The relationship with birth

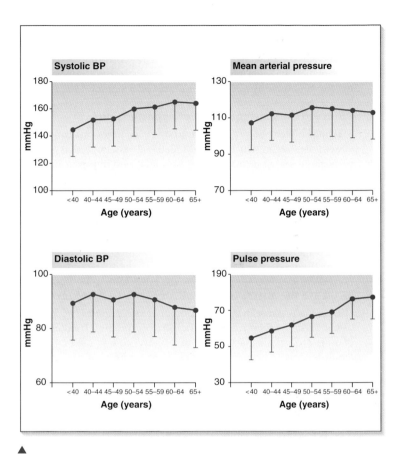

Fig. 1.3 Age and blood pressure. Age-related trends in systolic blood pressure, diastolic blood pressure, mean arterial pressure and pulse pressure for each 5-year age group from < 40 to > 65 years. (From Khattar *et al* 2001, with permission of the American Heart Association.)

weight has led to the concept of 'fetal programming' of blood pressure, where the influence of environmental factors during fetal development can predict subsequent blood pressure and cardiovascular disease risk.

CONSEQUENCES OF HYPERTENSION

1.12　Is hypertension an asymptomatic disease?

In the majority of patients, hypertension is a silent disease that can remain undetected for many years. Occasionally, headache can occur, particularly when the systolic blood pressure is elevated beyond 200 mmHg, or when blood pressure is rising rapidly, as can occur in malignant hypertension. In most cases, therefore, hypertension is diagnosed on routine blood pressure examination, or when a major complication arises. Nevertheless, malignant hypertension is associated with a number of symptoms (*Box 1.1*).

1.13 What are the consequences of hypertension?

Sustained high blood pressure progressively damages small and large blood vessels, resulting in structural and functional vessel wall changes. These pathognomonic abnormalities are associated with impaired autoregulation of blood flow, altered vessel wall shear stresses, and disrupted capillary permeability. Hypertension characteristically increases cardiac workload, resulting in progressive left ventricular hypertrophy and impaired myocardial perfusion, which predispose to myocardial ischaemia and cardiac failure. The consequences of hypertension manifest predominantly in the cardiovascular, cerebrovascular, and renovascular systems, as summarized in Box 1.2.

1.14 What are the absolute risks attributable to hypertension?

High blood pressure makes a significant contribution to an individual's overall cardiovascular risk. It must, therefore, be considered in the context of other predisposing factors, including advancing age, strongly positive family history, and coexistent independent cardiovascular risk factors, e.g.

BOX 1.2 Consequences of hypertension

Cardiac disease
- Left ventricular failure
- Angina
- Myocardial infarction

Cerebrovascular disease
- Transient ischaemic attacks
- Stroke
- Multi-infarct dementia
- Hypertensive encephalopathy

Vascular
- Aortic aneurysm
- Occlusive peripheral vascular disease

Others
- Progressive renal failure
- Hypertensive retinopathy

TABLE 1.2 Relative risk of hypertension and other selected factors in predicting future stroke

Risk factor	Relative risk
Hypertension	7.0
Cardiac disease	3.0
Left ventricular hypertrophy	4.4
Atrial fibrillation	3.7
Previous transient ischaemic attack	5–13
Diabetes: male	4.1
Diabetes: female	5.8

diabetes mellitus, smoking and hypercholesterolaemia. Multivariate analysis has been used to determine the particular contribution made by high blood pressure to overall cardiovascular risk, and it appears that hypertension is one of the most significant single, modifiable risk factors. For example, in western populations, hypertension confers up to a sevenfold increase in the risk of stroke (*Table 1.2*). Furthermore, hypertension is thought to account for one-half of all deaths due to stroke, and up to one-quarter of coronary heart disease deaths. Consequently, there are potentially very substantial opportunities for reducing cardiovascular morbidity and mortality by appropriate identification and management of individuals with raised blood pressure (Rodgers *et al* 2000, Rudd *et al* 1997).

1.15 Is the relationship between blood pressure and risk continuous?

There is an association between advancing age and the prevalence of hypertension, and the incidence of cardiovascular disease, particularly stroke and coronary heart disease, progressively increases with age. Importantly, the relationship between raised blood pressure and cardiovascular disease risk persists, regardless of age. Hypertension confers increased cardiovascular risk at all ages, and should not be viewed as a normal part of ageing. Furthermore, the relationship between blood pressure and risk appears to be linear and it is, therefore, difficult to define a normal reference range for blood pressure on the basis of cardiovascular risk alone (*Figs 1.4 and 1.5*).

1.16 Is there a J-shaped curve?

There has been controversy surrounding the possibility of a J-curve relation between blood pressure and cardiovascular mortality. Observational data from the Framingham Study indicate a very clear relationship between rising blood pressure and cardiovascular mortality risk. Controversially, the lowest blood pressure decile is not associated with lowest overall risk

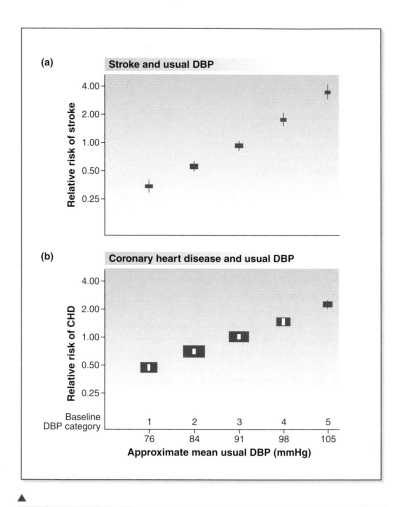

▲

Fig. 1.4 Blood pressure and relative risk of stroke and coronary heart disease. **A.** Stroke and usual diastolic blood pressure (DBP) (in five categories defined by baseline DBP) in 7 prospective observational studies: 843 events. **B.** Coronary heart disease and usual DBP (in five categories defined by baseline DBP) in 9 prospective observational studies: 4856 events. (From McMahon *et al* 1990 with permission.)

(*Fig. 1.6*), and this has suggested that some critical blood pressure level may be required to prevent harm, perhaps by maintaining adequate coronary artery perfusion. However, these observational data are heavily confounded by inclusion of individuals who have low blood pressure as a manifestation

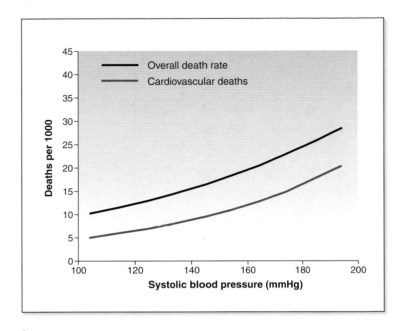

Fig. 1.5 Age-adjusted cardiovascular mortality and systolic blood pressure in the Framingham study population. (From Port *et al* 2000 with permission.)

of cardiovascular or other diseases, and who would, therefore, be more predisposed to an adverse outcome. The consensus view supports the epidemiological finding of a linear relation between blood pressure and cardiovascular risk, with no definitive evidence of a lower limit below which risk increases. Furthermore, clinical trials of hypertension treatment have failed to demonstrate optimal systolic and diastolic blood pressure targets, where benefits are attenuated by further blood pressure lowering.

1.17 Does white-coat hypertension carry a risk?

In the past, 'white-coat' hypertension was thought to be an innocent phenomenon, partly because of the apparently short-lived nature of the blood pressure increase in the setting of situational stress or anxiety. However, early clinical trials showing benefits from blood pressure lowering enrolled patients on the basis of serial office recordings and, therefore, were likely to have included patients with white-coat hypertension. The clinical significance of white-coat hypertension is controversial, and several studies indicate a higher prevalence of metabolic abnormalities consistent with the insulin resistance syndrome, possibly mediated by increased sympathetic

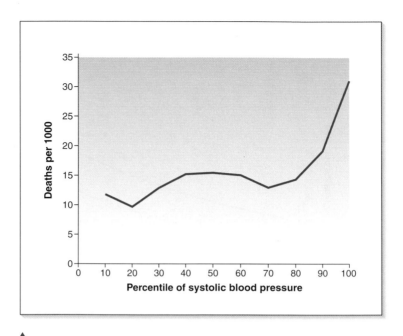

▲

Fig. 1.6 Cardiovascular mortality in the Framingham study population by systolic blood pressure centile. (From Port *et al* 2000 with permission.)

adrenergic activity. Target organ damage and cardiovascular mortality risk lies between that of normotensives and individuals with sustained hypertension. Furthermore, individuals with white-coat hypertension or abnormally variable blood pressure are at increased risk of sustained hypertension. In a 5-year follow-up study of healthy army personnel the risk of future hypertension among individuals with transient hypertension at outset was three to six times higher than among normotensives. In view of the increased risk associated with white-coat hypertension, antihypertensive treatment should be considered appropriate in the majority of cases.

1.18 What is the risk of malignant hypertension?

Malignant hypertension remains one of the immediate life-threatening complications of blood pressure elevation and is associated with a variety of end-organ damage (*Table 1.3*). Cerebral blood flow is autoregulated within specific limits, and normally cerebral blood flow remains unchanged between mean arterial pressures of 60 mmHg and 120 mmHg. As mean arterial pressure increases, compensatory cerebral vasoconstriction limits

TABLE 1.3 Consequences of malignant hypertension	
End organ	**Complications**
Aorta	Aortic dissection
Brain	Hypertensive encephalopathy
	Cerebral infarction or haemorrhage
Heart	Cardiac failure
	Myocardial ischaemia/infarction
Kidney	Renal failure
Placenta	Eclampsia

cerebral hyperperfusion, but beyond a mean arterial pressure of about 180 mmHg this autoregulation is overwhelmed and cerebral vasodilatation and oedema ensue. Previously normotensive individuals can develop signs of encephalopathy at blood pressures as low as 160/100 mmHg, whereas individuals with long-standing hypertension may not do so until the blood pressure rises to 220/110 mmHg or greater. Untreated, the 5-year mortality approaches 100%, but is dramatically reduced by pharmacological intervention. However, blood pressure should be reduced gradually in the majority of cases apart from true 'hypertensive emergencies' such as encephalopathy, acute left ventricular failure and aortic dissection.

1.19 What is the risk of isolated systolic hypertension?

Isolated systolic hypertension increases the risk of stroke and coronary heart disease by ~40%, and cardiovascular death by ~50%. It is also associated with an increase of ~50% in the development of heart failure in older individuals.

1.20 Is systolic or diastolic blood pressure more important?

The latest data from the Framingham Heart Study in particular suggest that diastolic blood pressure is the best predictor of coronary heart risk in the under 50s; that both systolic and diastolic pressures are equally predictive in the 50–60 age range; and that after 60 years of age systolic and pulse pressure become dominant. Indeed, in the over-50s for any given systolic pressure the *lower* the diastolic pressure the *higher* the risk of coronary heart disease. However, when assessing risk it is important to take both values into consideration. In particular, marked elevation of either systolic or diastolic pressure should not be ignored, even if the other parameter is 'normal'. Therefore, a 65-year-old with a blood pressure of 154/120 mmHg should still be treated because of the marked diastolic pressure elevation.

PATIENT QUESTIONS

1.21 What is hypertension?

Hypertension simply means raised, or high, blood pressure. Blood pressure depends on how much blood the heart pumps out each minute and on the resistance to blood flow, which is controlled by the tiny blood vessels. Most hypertension is the result of an increase in the resistance to blood flow because of changes in these blood vessels. However, what causes this is still unknown and doctors call this form of high blood pressure 'essential hypertension'. In a small number of cases (less than 1 in 10), a cause for the high blood pressure can be identified, and this is called 'secondary hypertension'.

1.22 What do the two numbers mean?

Blood pressure is usually quoted as two numbers. These are written as 120/80 (said '120 over 80'). The measurement units are millimetres of mercury, which is abbreviated to 'mmHg', and come from the fact that blood pressure is traditionally measured with a mercury sphygmomanometer. The top number refers to 'systolic pressure', which is the maximum pressure per heart beat, and the bottom to 'diastolic' pressure, which is the minimum value. Elevation of either number can imply hypertension, and both are probably equally important.

1.23 What level of blood pressure is high?

Blood pressure varies second-by-second and from day to day. There is also a large variation in blood pressure within the population – just like height. Therefore, there is no simple definition of hypertension. However, to guide doctors several authorities have set a level of less than 140/90 mmHg as normal and over 160/100 mmHg as high and thus requiring therapy. Between the two is a grey area, and other factors such as smoking and cholesterol will determine whether blood pressure should be lowered.

1.24 Is high blood pressure bad for you?

Sustained high blood pressure is associated with an increase in the risk of strokes, heart attacks, heart failure and death: the higher the pressure the more the risk. However, lowering blood pressure with drugs and other means reduces this risk and improves life expectancy. Rarely, blood pressure can cause confusion, coma and visual problems, and this may require emergency treatment.

1.25 What is a stroke?

A stroke occurs when part of the brain is starved of blood and as a result dies. The cells that make up the brain cannot regenerate, so often some function of the brain – such as movement of a hand, or speech – is lost. However, as the associated swelling reduces and other parts of the brain take over some of the functions of the damaged area there is often some recovery, which can be almost full. Strokes are usually caused by blockage of an artery or bleeding into the brain. High blood pressure is a risk factor for both types of stroke.

1.26 Does hypertension cause symptoms?

In most people hypertension does not produce any symptoms, hence the importance of regular blood pressure checks. Indeed, hypertension has been called 'the silent killer'. Although many people believe that high blood pressure causes headaches, this is untrue except in a very small number of people with very high blood pressure. In fact, in carefully controlled studies, headache is equally common in people with high and normal blood pressure. Very rarely, high blood pressure may cause problems with vision, breathlessness, confusion, and even coma.

Aetiology of primary hypertension

2

ESSENTIAL HYPERTENSION

2.1 How is blood pressure regulated?

Systemic blood pressure is determined by the cardiac output and total peripheral vascular resistance (*Box 2.1*), and is closely regulated by several integrated physiological mechanisms. In particular, sympathetic neural and hormonal activity, increase cardiac output and systemic vascular resistance, leading to a rise in blood pressure, which is augmented to some extent by activation of the renin–angiotensin–aldosterone system. These effects are opposed by the direct cardiac influence of the parasympathetic limb of the autonomic nervous system. Furthermore, the resistance blood vessels themselves play a crucial role in maintaining normal blood pressure through the production and release of the vasodilator, nitric oxide, which reduces systemic vascular resistance.

The baroreflex contributes to short-term regulation of blood pressure. Blood pressure is 'sensed' by specialized stretch receptors (baroreceptors) in the walls of the aortic arch and the carotid blood vessels. Baroreceptor firing rate during each systolic pulsation is proportional to blood pressure, and conveyed via afferent fibres to a central blood pressure regulatory site, which in turn determines the degree of sympathetic and parasympathetic outflow to the heart and blood vessels. Therefore, in health, the baroreflex mechanism maintains beat-to-beat blood pressure homeostasis, principally mediated through the autonomic nervous system.

2.2 What is the physiological basis of essential hypertension?

The exact physiological basis of essential hypertension remains uncertain. Our understanding of the mechanisms involved in its pathogenesis has increased substantially, and it has also become clear that both genetic and environmental factors can contribute. Essential hypertension is associated with elevated systolic and diastolic blood pressure, and usually accompanied by increased systemic vascular resistance, at least in its established phase. The arterial wall in hypertension is characterized by medial thickening due to smooth muscle proliferation. It is unclear whether these changes are primary or secondary but they will, in either case, exacerbate hypertension through further increases in systemic vascular resistance, owing to attenuation of arteriolar surface area.

A further characteristic feature of essential hypertension is resetting of baroreceptor sensitivity to changes in blood pressure, possibly as a

---

BOX 2.1 Haemodynamics

Mean arterial pressure = Cardiac output × Peripheral vascular resistance

Pulse pressure ∝ Cardiac output, Arterial compliance, Wave reflection consequence of arteriolar medial hyperplasia. Increased systemic vascular resistance and impaired baroreflex sensitivity are important maladaptive responses that beget further increases in blood pressure.

2.3   Does the sympathetic nervous system play a role?

There is mounting evidence that increased sympathetic tone, and decreased parasympathetic tone, make a substantial contribution to essential hypertension, particularly in younger patients with early, 'borderline' hypertension. Total brain, and in particular subcortical, turnover of noradrenaline (norepinephrine) is substantially higher in hypertensive than in normotensive individuals. Heart rate variability is largely determined by sympathetic (low-frequency variability) and parasympathetic (high-frequency variability) activity, and both frequency components can be determined by power spectral analysis of continuous ECG recordings. This technique has provided evidence of increased sympathetic and decreased parasympathetic cardiac influence. Microneurography of sympathetic fibres carried by the common peroneal nerve has provided direct evidence of increased sympathetic neuronal outflow in young hypertensives. Therefore, a large body of evidence, both direct and indirect, suggests that excess sympathetic activity is an important mechanism in essential hypertension, particularly in younger patient groups.

2.4   Is the kidney involved in the genesis of essential hypertension?

The renin–angiotensin system is an integrated hormonal cascade that is responsible for control of renal function, blood pressure, and fluid and electrolyte balance. Renin is secreted by the macula densa in the juxtaglomerular apparatus, adjacent to the afferent arteriole of the nephron, in response to reduced renal blood flow. Renin acts on angiotensinogen to form angiotensin I, which is in turn converted to angiotensin II by angiotensin-converting enzyme (ACE). Angiotensin II is a potent vasoconstrictor, and stimulus for aldosterone release from the adrenal cortex, which enhances renal salt and water retention (*Fig. 2.1*). The renin–angiotensin system, therefore, serves to maintain blood pressure in situations where renal blood flow or blood volume is significantly reduced, and is comparatively quiescent in healthy, well-hydrated individuals. However, in ~15% of hypertensives there is significantly, and inappropriately, elevated plasma renin activity, suggesting that the renin–angiotensin system may play an important role in elevating blood pressure in these individuals. Furthermore, these patients show a particularly effective blood pressure reduction in response to renin–angiotensin system blockade by ACE inhibitors or angiotensin-receptor antagonist drugs. Therefore, excessive renin–angiotensin system

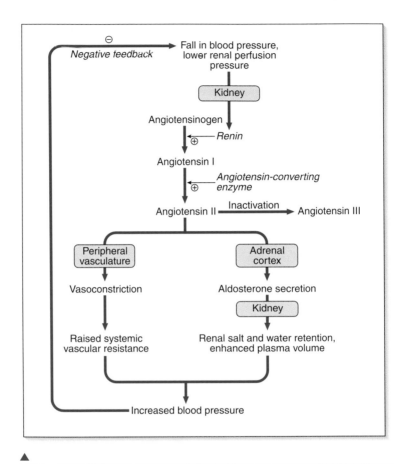

Fig. 2.1 The role of the renin–angiotensin–aldosterone system (RAAS) in physiological regulation of blood pressure.

activation appears to contribute to the development of hypertension, and this is particularly evident in a small subgroup of patients.

2.5   Is there a genetic predisposition to hypertension?

The role for a genetic contribution to the development of hypertension has become apparent from studies of communities, families and twins, and the identification and localization of specific genes for hypertension is currently underway. Several gene loci have been described for important, albeit rare forms of hypertension. For example, the autosomal-dominant hypertensive syndrome of glucocorticoid-remediable hyperaldosteronism (*see* Qs 9.57) has been shown to result from a genetic chimerism of the genes encoding 11β-hydroxylase and aldosterone synthase. The gene for angiotensinogen has been associated with essential hypertension and hypertension in pregnancy, although the clinical significance of this remains unclear. The search for candidate genes that contribute to hypertension is a huge challenge, made particularly difficult by heterogeneity of the phenotype. Identification may be facilitated by restricting the study population to a particular phenotypic subtype, based, for example, on plasma renin activity or membrane channel transporters characteristics. Where single or multiple genes contribute to hypertension, these are likely to act by rendering individuals more susceptible to environmental influences, such that the interaction between genes and other factors is likely to have a significant influence.

ISOLATED SYSTOLIC HYPERTENSION

2.6   What is isolated systolic hypertension?

Isolated systolic hypertension refers to the situation of a raised systolic pressure in conjunction with a normal or even low diastolic pressure, i.e. a widened pulse pressure. Once again definitions are purely arbitrary (*Box 2.2*) but from a practical point of view in the UK the British Hypertension Society (BHS) guidelines are used, and in the USA the criteria laid down by the Sixth Joint National Committee (JNC VI). Isolated systolic hypertension is a common disorder in western countries, especially in older individuals. Indeed, using the BHS definition it is estimated that it affects ~25% of those aged over 60 years, but over 50% if the JNC VI criteria are applied. In contrast, isolated systolic hypertension is uncommon in those aged under 50 years (*Fig. 2.2*).

2.7   What is the pathophysiological basis of isolated systolic hypertension?

Isolated systolic hypertension results from stiffening of the large arteries, and in contrast to 'classical' essential hypertension in young and middle-aged subjects, is not primarily associated with an increase in peripheral

---

BOX 2.2   Defining isolated systolic hypertension

British Hypertension Society
Systolic ≥160 and diastolic <90 mmHg

Joint National Committee
Systolic ≥140 and diastolic <90 mmHg

World Health Authority–International Society of Hypertension
Systolic ≥140 and diastolic <90 mmHg

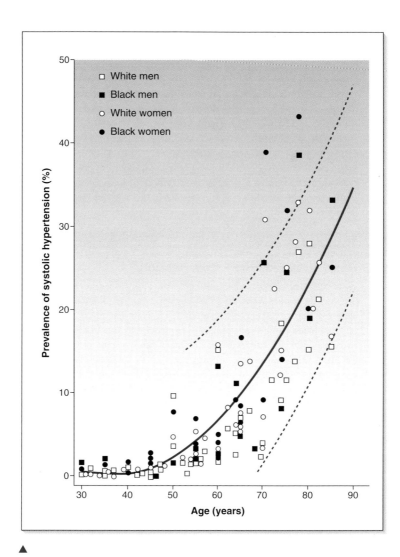

▲

Fig. 2.2 The prevalence of isolated systolic hypertension by age: data from various studies. (From Staessen J, Amery A, Fagard R 1990 Isolated systolic hypertension in the elderly. Journal of Hypertension 8:393–405, with permission of Lippincott, Williams & Wilkins.)

vascular resistance (*Box 2.1*). In almost all populations there is an age-related increase in large artery stiffness. This is thought to be due to disruption and disorganization of elastic elements (mainly elastin and collagen) within the arterial wall, which results in dilatation and stiffening of the artery – the process of arteriosclerosis (not to be confused with atherosclerosis). Certain conditions such as diabetes and hypertension itself are thought to accelerate this phenomenon and thus predispose to systolic hypertension. However, isolated systolic hypertension is not the 'burnt-out' phase of diastolic hypertension, as fewer than 20% of subjects with isolated systolic hypertension have had diastolic hypertension previously documented (Bulpitt *et al* 1995). Importantly, isolated systolic hypertension is not a benign condition and is associated with considerable excess cardiovascular morbidity and mortality (*see Q. 1.19*).

2.8 Will everyone develop isolated systolic hypertension?

Isolated systolic hypertension can be viewed as an exaggeration of the 'normal' age-related increase in arterial stiffness. Alternatively, one may consider it something we might all develop should we live long enough! Interestingly, data from the Framingham Study (Franklin *et al* 1997) suggest that individuals with a slightly higher pulse pressure aged 30–40 have an accelerated widening of pulse pressure with age and, therefore, the 'seeds' of isolated systolic hypertension may be set many years before the condition becomes manifest.

2.9 Can we reverse isolated systolic hypertension?

At present, the mainstay of therapy for isolated systolic hypertension is traditional antihypertensive drugs, which are mainly targeted to reduce peripheral vascular resistance and/or cardiac output. Nevertheless, by reducing mean blood pressure the large arteries become less stiff and pulse pressure is reduced, i.e. systolic pressure tends to be lowered more than diastolic pressure. Indeed, calcium-channel blockers and thiazide diuretic both reduce cardiovascular events in subjects with isolated systolic hypertension (*see Ch. 7*). However, there is considerable interest in developing drugs specifically targeted at the large arteries, acting either on smooth muscle, such as nitric oxide donors, or to 'repair' the disrupted elastin and collagen fibres.

2.10 Can we prevent isolated systolic hypertension?

At present, there are no specific therapies designed to prevent the development of isolated systolic hypertension. However, it is likely that aggressive control of cardiovascular risk factors, the majority of which also promote arterial stiffening, may reduce the risk of systolic hypertension in later life.

LIFESTYLE FACTORS CAUSING HYPERTENSION

2.11 Does being overweight predispose to high blood pressure?

Epidemiological studies demonstrate a clear association between hypertension and obesity. Moreover, obesity is a strong independent risk factor for the development of hypertension (Stamler et al 1978). Indeed, the prevalence of hypertension in the obese has been estimated to be between 50–300% higher than in lean subjects, and a recent Cochrane review suggested that 40% of hypertensives have coexisting obesity (Mulrow et al 2000). In addition body weight correlates with blood pressure within the 'normotensive' range (Hypertension Prevention Trial Research Group 1990), and some investigators have suggested that body fat distribution is a more powerful determinant of blood pressure than overall measures of obesity.

2.12 Is dietary salt intake important?

Dietary salt intake and its relationship to hypertension remains a contentious issue. The INTERSALT Study (Rose & Stamler 1989) analysed data from 10079 individuals recruited from 48 centres worldwide. It demonstrated a significant, positive association between 24-hour urinary sodium excretion, as a marker of salt intake, and systolic blood pressure. For both men and women the association between sodium and systolic pressure was stronger for the older than the younger adults. The association between salt and blood pressure is supported by numerous randomized trials showing that low-salt diets can produce significant reductions in blood pressure.

2.13 Does excess alcohol intake cause hypertension?

The INTERSALT Study (Marmot et al 1994) assessed the influence of alcohol intake on blood pressure in 4844 men and 4837 women aged between 20 and 59 who were recruited from 57 centres worldwide. The results demonstrated a clear and significant positive relationship between heavy drinking (3–4 or more drinks per day) and blood pressure in both men and women. The relationship was independent of, and added to, the effect on blood pressure of body mass index and urinary excretion of sodium. Acute alcohol consumption has also been demonstrated to increase blood pressure, but observational studies show an inverse relationship between coronary artery disease and alcohol consumption (Thun et al 1997). The relationship between alcohol consumption and blood pressure is generally a linear one.

PQ PATIENT QUESTIONS

2.14 Does high blood pressure run in families?

In some cases, high blood pressure does appear to run in families, and many people can often find a first-degree relative with hypertension. However, this is not always the case. In a very few cases we understand why blood pressure is inherited and scientists have identified the 'faulty' gene responsible. However, in the vast majority of cases no one gene seems responsible.

2.15 Should my children be screened for blood pressure?

Most high blood pressure only becomes apparent in adult life, and it is not generally recommended that blood pressure be assessed in all children. However, in families known to have some rare forms of hypertension, or in those in which hypertension has been previously discovered in children or adolescents, it is certainly worthwhile screening children for hypertension. In addition, adolescent females considering taking the oral contraceptive pill must have their blood pressure assessed regularly.

2.16 What is white-coat hypertension?

This term refers to the situation when a person's blood pressure is raised whilst visiting the doctor (hence 'white-coat') but is normal outside this setting. It is commonly diagnosed by measuring the blood pressure at the clinic and then for a period of 24 hours while in the home setting (called 'ambulatory blood pressure monitoring'). Alternatively, blood pressure may be assessed using an automatic machine at home. It is important to realize that everyone's blood pressure is lower when measured at home, even people with hypertension, and that an allowance must be made for this. Additionally, whether white-coat hypertension increases the risk of strokes and heart attacks, and thus requires treating, remains uncertain.

Clinical assessment in hypertension

3

HISTORY EXAMINATION AND INVESTIGATION

3.1 What symptoms are associated with essential hypertension?

The majority of patients with essential hypertension will be completely asymptomatic; therefore, detection will depend on routine measurement of blood pressure. However, those with malignant hypertension or secondary hypertension may experience symptoms such as headache (*see Q. 1.12*). The fact that hypertension is effectively a symptom-free disease has major implications for long-term management, because patients will not feel intrinsically better for having their blood pressure lowered. Therefore, drugs and non-pharmacological measures need to be well tolerated.

3.2 What are the features suggestive of secondary hypertension?

Idiopathic, or essential, hypertension accounts for more than 95% of cases, although in many cases aggravating factors, such as alcohol excess and obesity, can be identified. However, a cause can be identified in around 5–10% of patients with hypertension – so-called secondary hypertension (*see Ch. 9*). The accuracy of history and examination, in estimating the likelihood of a secondary cause of hypertension, has been poorly studied. Features suggesting an underlying renovascular cause include drug-resistant hypertension, hypertension onset beyond 60 years of age, flank bruit, and a significant rise in creatinine during ACE inhibitor treatment. Phaeochromocytoma may be suggested by a diverse range of clinical features including headache, palpitation, particularly labile blood pressure, and a paradoxical blood pressure increase with β-blocker therapy owing to unopposed intense α-receptor-mediated vasoconstriction. Persistent hypokalaemia may be due to underlying primary hyperaldosteronism.

Such clinical features may suggest a secondary cause for hypertension, and consideration should be given to further investigation. The enthusiasm with which a secondary cause is sought will depend on other factors, for example whether blood pressure control can be attained without the need for any further intervention, or whether the results of such investigation, e.g. renal artery stenosis, would result in intervention and alter treatment.

3.3 What are the key features of malignant hypertension?

Malignant, or accelerated, hypertension is a medical emergency characterized by severe hypertension, often due to rapid elevation of blood pressure, with evidence of end-organ damage. Focal cerebral oedema owing to loss of autoregulation results in hypertensive encephalopathy. The majority of encephalopathy patients present with headache, but in up to a third, delirium, hemiparesis, cortical visual loss or coma may occur. About 30% of patients with malignant hypertension present with cardiac failure and pulmonary oedema, owing to the combination of increased circulating volume, increased cardiac afterload, and functional impairment of the ischaemic left ventricle. Acute renal impairment occurs in the majority of patients with malignant hypertension, and is virtually always associated with increased circulating fluid volume. In severe cases, dialysis may be required, particularly when there is pre-existing renal disease, and the prognosis is better if renal size, assessed by ultrasonography, is normal. Microscopic appearances indicate renal ischaemia and acute tubular necrosis, along with characteristic features of hypertensive end-organ damage, including fibrinoid necrosis and hyaline arteriosclerosis. In some cases, malignant hypertension can be associated with abdominal pain due to gastrointestinal ischaemia, and even intestinal and pancreatic infarction.

3.4 What are the key points in the history?

On most occasions, hypertension will be detected during routine screening, and patients may not present with specific symptoms. It is important to establish the duration of hypertension where possible. Therefore, ask about the results of any previous blood pressure checks, for example attendance at an earlier clinic or insurance medical. The occurrence of hypertension during pregnancy should be noted, and any family history of hypertension and cardiovascular disease should be elicited. In order to address overall cardiovascular disease risk, other major risk factors should be sought including smoking habit, diabetes mellitus, and hypercholesterolaemia if known. Aggravating factors for hypertension should also be sought, including assessment of alcohol intake, levels of physical activity, and dietary habits such as salt intake, and fresh fruit and vegetable consumption. Finally, it is important to consider features that might suggest an underlying cause for high blood pressure. For example, headache, palpitation, and excessive sweatiness could suggest a phaeochromocytoma.

3.5 What are the key points to look for in the examination?

In addition to careful assessment of the blood pressure itself (*see Qs 3.17–3.24*), a full physical examination is required. It is important that height, weight and body mass index (BMI) are documented (BMI = weight ÷ [height]^2 (kg/m^2)). Cardiovascular system examination should focus on evidence of heart failure, cardiac arrhythmia and peripheral arterial insufficiency, whilst the kidneys should be examined carefully for apparent bruits or masses. Examination of the central nervous system should be performed, looking for any clinical signs of cerebrovascular damage, and the appearance of both retinas should be noted.

3.6   What is end-organ damage?

End-organ damage is a collective term used to describe a pattern of abnormalities that occur as a direct consequence of exposure to persistently high blood pressure. Resistance arterioles, exposed directly to increased wall tension and lumen pressure, undergo morphological changes, characterized by smooth muscle hypertrophy and collagen deposition in the subendothelial space, leading to the pathognomonic microscopic appearance known as hyaline arteriosclerosis. These structural changes reduce vessel lumen, thus increasing systemic vascular resistance, and hence high blood pressure begets further increased blood pressure.

Many organs are protected from the effects of elevated systemic blood pressure by autoregulation, which serves to maintain normal tissue blood flow, and when hypertension is slowly progressive there is a degree of adaptation to higher pressures. However, continuous exposure to elevated blood pressure ultimately leads to organ damage, and the most important clinical sites are the kidney, heart, and brain.

Hypertensive nephropathy is associated with a gradual decline in creatinine clearance, and in cases of malignant hypertension, acute renal failure can occur.

Cardiac end-organ response to sustained hypertension is concentric left ventricular hypertrophy, which may be detected by electrocardiography (*Fig. 3.1*) or, in some cases, by echocardiography. Together with an altered perfusion gradient because of higher ventricular pressure, this places increased demand on coronary blood supply, and predisposes to myocardial ischaemia and microscopic foci of myocardial necrosis, which further impair cardiac performance. Left ventricular hypertrophy is a poor prognostic indicator in hypertensive patients, irrespective of blood pressure itself, and may regress if adequate blood pressure control is attained.

Disruption of normal cerebral blood flow often manifests insidiously, and predisposes to progressive cortical loss, manifesting as non-Alzheimer's dementia. In malignant hypertension, rapid elevation of blood pressure can overwhelm cerebral autoregulation mechanisms, typically where mean arterial pressure exceeds 180 mmHg. This can cause cerebral arteriolar vasodilatation, oedema, and microhaemorrhages, presenting clinically as delirium or acute encephalopathy (hypertensive encephalopathy).

3.7   How is hypertensive retinopathy graded?

Hypertensive retinopathy reflects the abnormal microvascular responses to hypertension occurring elsewhere in the body. The features of hypertensive

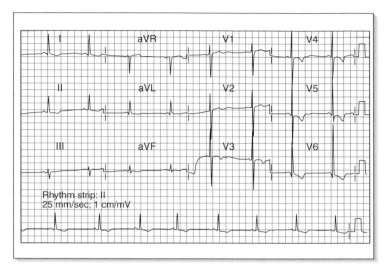

▲

Fig. 3.1 Typical ECG features of left ventricular hypertrophy (LVH) with 'strain' pattern in the lateral leads: 'S' in V2 + 'R' in V5 >35 mm; 'S-T' depression and inverted 'T' waves in V3–V6, I and aVL.

retinopathy can include the appearance of cotton wool spots, flame-shaped haemorrhages, macular oedema, macular star/ring of exudates, disc oedema, and ultimately papilloedema (*Fig. 3.2*). Exudation and papilloedema are thought to arise from accumulation of axoplasmatic debris due to ischaemia-induced obstruction of axoplasmic flow. The severity of hypertensive retinopathy can be described by several grading systems, and that endorsed by the British Hypertension Society, is the Keith, Wagener and Barker classification (*Table 3.1*).

3.8 What is the significance of proteinuria?

Proteinuria is a very sensitive marker of early hypertensive renal damage, and is often associated with elevated serum urea and creatinine concentrations. Its presence is indicative of worsened prognosis and, together with raised serum urea and creatinine, predicts increased mortality in accelerated hypertension, owing to renal failure, stroke, myocardial infarction and heart failure (Lip *et al* 1995, Weinstock & Keane 2001). Established microalbuminuria is an independent risk factor for progression of renal disease in hypertensive patients, and reduction of proteinuria by ACE-inhibitor treatment has been associated with delayed decline of renal function.

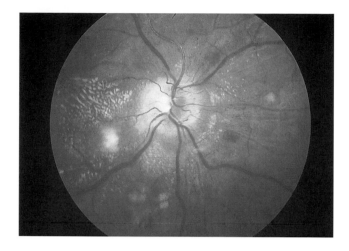

▲

Fig. 3.2 Hypertensive retinopathy. Fundus from a 24-year-old woman with malignant hypertension, illustrating grade VI retinopathy. Note the presence of papilloedema cotton wool spots, and haemorrhages.

TABLE 3.1 Grades of hypertensive retinopathy

Grade	Features
Grade I	Mild narrowing or sclerosis of the retinal arterioles No symptoms; good general health
Grade II	Moderate to marked sclerosis of the retinal arterioles Exaggerated light reflex Venous compression at arteriovenous crossings ('AV nipping') No symptoms; good general health
Grade III	Retinal oedema, cotton wool spots Haemorrhages Sclerosis and spastic lesions of retinal arterioles Often symptomatic
Grade IV (malignant hypertension)	All of the above Optic disc oedema (papilloedema) Symptomatic Cardiac and renal function often impaired; reduced survival

From Dodson *et al.* 1996, with permission of the Nature Publishing Group.

3.9 What is the significance of haematuria?

Microscopic haematuria is also a marker of hypertensive renal damage, although it is less closely related to clinical outcome than proteinuria. The renal morphological changes associated with essential hypertension include hyaline arteriosclerosis, focal glomerular obsolescence and thickening of glomerular basement membranes (Katz *et al* 1979). These renal abnormalities are associated with decreased glomerular filtration, red blood cell urinary casts, and in some cases persistent microscopic haematuria. Haematuria is also associated with some forms of renal parenchyma disease, and may therefore suggest an underlying cause for hypertension.

3.10 What laboratory investigations are required?

These are outlined in Box 3.1.

BOX 3.1 Routine and selected investigations in patients with hypertension

Routinely indicated
- Urinalysis for protein and blood
- Serum urea, creatinine and electrolytes
- Blood glucose
- Serum total:HDL cholesterol
- ECG

Indicated in selected patients
- Chest x-ray
- Urine microscopy and culture
- Echocardiography

3.11 Should lipids be assessed only in the fasting state?

The initial measurement of random (non-fasting) total cholesterol and HDL cholesterol can be used as a screen to estimate an individual's coronary heart disease risk. However, this may need to be repeated in the fasting state, in order to more accurately determine total:HDL cholesterol ratio, and whether drug therapy is indicated in some individuals.

3.12 Should uric acid be measured?

Uric acid is not measured consistently in the assessment of all hypertensive patients, largely because debate persists as to whether raised serum urate is an independent cardiovascular risk factor, or simply a marker of other factors. However, raised serum urate concentrations can demarcate

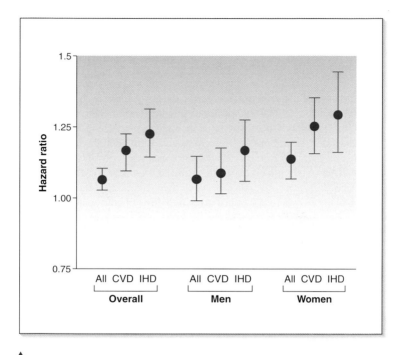

Fig. 3.3 Serum urate and cardiovascular risk. Hazard ratio for highest compared to lowest quartile of serum urate concentration for all-cause, cardiovascular and ischaemic heart disease mortality risk in males, females and the whole population that participated in the First National Health and Nutrition Examination Survey, 1971–75. (From Fang & Alderman 2000, with permission of the American Medical Association.)

individuals (*Fig. 3.3*) at particularly high risk of subsequent cardiovascular events, including stroke, and may, therefore, provide useful information for further risk stratification of hypertensive patients alongside that obtained from measuring conventional, established risk factors (Waring *et al* 2000). Routine measurement of serum urate concentrations may also be important in identifying those patients with particularly high concentrations who may be exposed to a greater risk of gout, especially if thiazide diuretic treatment is contemplated.

3.13 Do all patients need an ECG?

An ECG is recommended for all patients with hypertension. This serves as a crude screen for left ventricular hypertrophy, which is an important independent risk factor in hypertensive patients. Moreover, a routine ECG will rule out any underlying cardiac dysrhythmia, and in some cases can identify coexistent myocardial ischaemia.

3.14 Who needs an echocardiogram?

An echocardiogram (ECHO) is most useful for confirming or refuting the presence of left ventricular hypertrophy (LVH), where there is some degree of suspicion. LVH is an important independent marker of increased cardiovascular risk in hypertension, and the presence of LVH may be suggested by findings on physical examination, including left parasternal heave, chest X-ray, or on the ECG, for example high left ventricular voltages, S-T segment depression, and dysrhythmia. In addition, echocardiography is indicated when there is evidence of target organ damage elsewhere, for example retinopathy or nephropathy.

3.15 Who needs a chest X-ray?

A chest X-ray is not part of routine assessment of hypertensive patients. Rather it is reserved for those patients in whom symptoms or physical signs suggest involvement of the respiratory system, particularly where pulmonary oedema is suspected.

3.16 How should secondary causes of hypertension be excluded?

In evaluation of the hypertensive patient, patient characteristics, symptoms and/or physical signs, laboratory investigations, and response to treatment, may all suggest an underlying cause (*Table 3.2*). The nature of any further investigations will be directed by the suspected underlying cause and, in most cases, these will require specialist referral.

MEASURING BLOOD PRESSURE

3.17 How should blood pressure be measured?

Usually, blood pressure is measured in the brachial artery after 5 minutes' seated rest. It is important to use the correct size of cuff – the bladder should enclose 80% of the arm. The cuff should be applied securely to the upper arm, with the bladder centred over the brachial artery; further details of the manual technique are given in Box 3.2. Usually at least two measurements should be taken, and if they vary widely, a third. The patient should be relaxed and comfortable, and should not talk whilst blood pressure is being assessed. Blood pressure should be recorded to the nearest 2 mmHg to avoid digit preference.

TABLE 3.2 Features suggestive of secondary hypertension

Cause	Suggestive features	Specialist investigations
Renovascular disease	Elderly, male, smoker Widespread atherosclerosis Hyperkalaemia or rise in creatinine in response to ACE-I	Renal artery angiography
Cushing's syndrome	Cushingoid appearance Muscle weakness, fatigue Hirsutism	Dexamethasone suppression test CT/MRI scan abdomen ± chest
Primary aldosteronism	Spontaneous hypokalaemia Diuretic-induced hypokalaemia Family history	Erect and supine aldosterone:plasma renin activity ratio Salt load and 24-h urine aldosterone
Phaeochromocytoma	Anxiety symptoms, tachycardia Postural hypotension Episodic headache	Plasma catecholamines 24-h urinary catecholamines MIBG uptake scintigraphy

---

BOX 3.2 Measuring blood pressure

The arm should be supported and held horizontal at the level of the mid-sternum. The cuff should be inflated whilst palpating the brachial artery until the pulse disappears. This provides an estimate of systolic pressure and ensures that the cuff is correctly seated on the arm. Deflate the cuff, and reinflate to 30 mmHg above estimated systolic pressure. Deflate at 2–3 mmHg per second and listen over the brachial artery for the first occurrence of repetitive tapping sounds (Korotkoff I), which equates to systolic pressure. Diastolic pressure is conventionally taken at the disappearance of sounds (Korotkoff V). If the sounds do not disappear, as is occasionally the case, e.g. in some pregnant women, muffling of the sounds (Korotkoff IV) is taken instead – this should be noted.

Full details are available from http://w3.abdn.ac.uk/BHS/booklet/proced.htm.

3.18 What about obese subjects and children?

It is important to realize that unless the correct size of cuff is used, blood pressure recordings will be inaccurate. Although using a cuff that is too large has little or no effect on measured blood pressure, using a cuff that is too small (i.e. the bladder does not encompass 80% of the arm) leads to an overestimation of blood pressure. Indeed, the most frequent cause of incorrect blood pressure measurement is an inappropriately small cuff – if in doubt use a larger cuff. Therefore, larger cuffs may well be required for obese subjects, and small cuffs are available for use in children.

3.19 Are automated sphygmomanometers to be preferred?

There are two basic types of automated sphygmomanometers – oscillometric and auscultatory. The former are much more commonly used in clinical practice and at home by patients. They rely on oscillations in the bladder induced by blood pulsating through a partly occluded brachial artery to estimate blood pressure (maximal oscillation occurs when cuff pressure equals brachial artery mean pressure). Although often easier to use, there is no real advantage to automated sphygmomanometers over traditional mercury column devices in everyday clinical practice, if appropriate training has been given. Nevertheless, automated devices do remove digit preference and provide a degree of measurement standardization, and are thus often used in the clinical trial setting. Importantly, oscillometric sphygmomanometers are thought to be less reliable in the elderly, and in patients with atrial fibrillation. However, only devices validated by the British Hypertension Society should be used – a list may be found at the following address: http://www.hyp.ac.uk/bhsinfo/bpmindex.html

3.20 Should blood pressure be measured in both arms?

Blood pressure should be measured in both arms during the initial assessment of all hypertensive patients. This is of particular importance when the clinical history suggests coarctation or other serious aortic pathology (e.g. dissection). However, in general, it does not matter which arm blood pressure is measured in, so long as pressure does not differ greatly between the two arms (<15 mmHg). If there is a significant difference, then the arm with the higher reading should be used and this noted.

3.21 Are lying and standing blood pressures required?

Blood pressure should be measured lying and after a brief period of standing (~60 seconds) at least once. If there is no significant drop (<15 mmHg), then this need only be repeated if symptoms suggest postural hypotension, which is more common in the elderly and those taking vasodilating agents such as α-blockers.

3.22 How many times should pressure be measured to establish a diagnosis of hypertension?

Conventionally, the minimum requirement would be two readings on three separate occasions spaced by about 1 month apart. However, in subjects with 'high normal' values, blood pressure may be observed for a longer period, although recent evidence suggests that such individuals are very likely to develop sustained hypertension. Conversely, the period of observation should be reduced in subjects with clear evidence of end-organ damage or accelerated (malignant) hypertension, so that treatment can be initiated sooner.

3.23 Is ambulatory blood pressure monitoring worthwhile?

Ambulatory blood pressure monitoring (ABPM) is not necessary for either diagnosis or management in the majority of hypertensive patients. Indeed, the risk associated with hypertension and benefits of therapy have been established using seated clinic pressure recordings (*see Q. 1.14*). However, ABPM can be useful in a few patients, such as those with particularly labile pressures and subjects with high clinic recordings but no evidence of end-organ damage. Importantly, average ABPM values are invariably lower that those recorded in the clinic and thus an individual with a daytime ABPM average of 150/100 mmHg is probably at more risk than a subject with the same clinic pressure. Therefore, thresholds for therapy and targets need to be lowered when ABPM values are used (~12/7 mmHg lower). Usually, the average daytime value is used from ABPM to guide management decisions. However, it has been suggested that the lack of a nocturnal 'dip' in blood pressure may be of prognostic significance.

3.24 Is home monitoring of blood pressure reliable?

Provided that the patient is correctly using a well-maintained, validated automated sphygmomanometer, then home monitoring is generally reliable. Indeed, home monitoring can shorten the time taken for diagnosis and to achieve target pressure once therapy has been initiated. However, as with ambulatory monitoring, home values are invariably lower that those obtained in the clinic and thresholds should be adjusted accordingly.

ROLE OF THE GP CLINIC AND PRACTICE NURSE

3.25 Should clinic nurses or doctors assess blood pressure?

In the setting of general practice, it is often better for routine blood pressure checks and follow-up visits to be performed by the practice nurse. This is especially true if the nurse has received training in the measurement of blood pressure (a training video is available from the British Hypertension Society web site: http://w3.abdn.ac.uk/BHS/booklet/proced.htm). Use of a practice nurse may also serve to minimize any 'white-coat' effect. Indeed, the National Service Frameworks for England and Wales both emphasize the importance and utility of nurse-led, doctor-supported clinics for the management of hypertension and also cardiovascular disease prevention. This is undoubtedly how hypertension will be managed in the future but will necessitate adequate financial investment in training and validation of nurses who will run such clinics.

3.26 Can patients be managed in general practice?

Ideally, the majority of hypertensive patients should be managed in general practice. However, to date, the management of hypertension both in the hospital and general practice setting has been suboptimal. This situation can be improved in a number of ways (*Box 3.3*).

3.27 Who should be referred to the specialist hypertension clinic?

Ideally, every hypertensive patient should be seen at least once by a specialist in hypertension. However, this is currently impractical, as there are very few hypertension specialists and indeed few specialist clinics. Thus, currently, any hypertensive patient who is referred may be seen in a variety

---

BOX 3.3 Effective management of hypertension in general practice

1. Adequate training and validation of practice nurses, including continuing education.
2. Adequate protocols for screening high-risk individuals to improve detection of hypertension.
3. Dissemination of national, international and local guidelines in terms of treatment thresholds and target values (including high-risk groups such as diabetics).
4. Hand-held patient record cards with accurate details of BP targets and drug therapy. Such cards should be regularly and clearly updated.
5. Every hypertensive patient should be assessed as to his or her 10-year absolute risk of a cardiovascular event. This will involve management of coexisting risk factors including age, sex, family history, previous cardiovascular disease, smoking, cholesterol, BMI and diabetes.
6. Better patient education and empowerment.

of specialist outpatient clinics including cardiology, nephrology, geriatrics, neurology or general medicine. This situation is clearly less than adequate. Although, as stated previously, the majority of patients can and should be managed in general practice, there are a number of compelling indications for specialist referral (*see Box 7.2*).

3.28 Are nurse-led hypertension clinics practical?

Not only are nurse-led, doctor-supported hypertension clinics practical, they have been advocated and endorsed by the recent government National Service Framework. Indeed, such clinics are now established and have demonstrated a high degree of patient compliance and satisfaction (Hall *et al* 2001). However, to be successful in the long term, they will need adequate resourcing and support from government.

For further information see
http://www.mrfc2000fsnet.co.uk

Guidelines

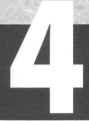

4.1 Why are guidelines needed?

Despite the clear evidence that the reduction of blood pressure is beneficial, treatment of hypertension remains suboptimal. Therefore, guidelines are needed in order to improve the treatment of hypertension in clinical practice. New evidence from observational and epidemiological studies, and randomized controlled trials is constantly emerging. The most recent British Hypertension Society (BHS) guidelines were published in 1999 (Ramsay *et al* 1999). Since the publication of the previous guidelines in 1993, new evidence has emerged on optimal blood pressure targets, management of hypertension in diabetics, treatment of isolated systolic hypertension in the elderly, and perhaps most contentiously the efficacy and tolerability of different classes of antihypertensive agent. The BHS guidelines categorized the strength of available evidence and the strength of their subsequent recommendations. Updates of World Health Organization (WHO)/International Society of Hypertension (ISH) guidelines will be posted here: http://www5.who.int/cardiovascular-diseases/

4.2 Why are there so many guidelines?

The large number of guidelines concerning hypertension reflect the constant stream of new information accruing from randomized controlled trials and also perhaps government policy in encouraging the practice of evidence-based medicine.

4.3 Which guideline should I follow?

It can be a difficult decision about which guideline to follow, given the increasing number of local and national guidelines currently available relating to hypertension. This is made worse by the sometimes contradictory nature of publications, such as the differing values of risk at which intervention should be initiated between the National Service Framework (NSF) and the Joint British Recommendations on Prevention of Coronary Heart Disease in Clinical Practice (British Cardiac Society *et al* 1998). However, this may relate more to economic considerations than evidence-based practice. What is most important is for clinics, general practitioners or local groups to decide for themselves which set of guidelines they wish to adopt, and then to make any modifications based upon local considerations. Indeed, local modification is something that the government seems likely to encourage in the near future.

4.4   How should guidelines be used?

Guidelines should be used to help established best evidence-based practice at a local level, taking into consideration the availability of resources, population demographics, and logistical factors. However, guidelines should be used to improve practice rather than criticize it.

4.5   What do the guidelines not cover?

The guidelines do not cover the practicalities and mechanics of implementation, especially relating to increased workloads and the need for additional resources. Indeed, if any of the current guidelines are to be implemented in full, considerable additional funding will be required. Since new risk factors are emerging continuously (e.g. serum homocysteine levels), guidelines date rapidly and will require frequent updating.

4.6   Do guidelines improve management?

The major reason behind the introduction of the guidelines by the BHS was to improve management of hypertension. Certainly, current guidelines do serve to draw doctors' and patients' attention to hypertension and modern trends in management. They may also assist in patient empowerment, which is likely to improve the number of patients reaching target values. Moreover, guidelines allow for internal and external audit, which hopefully can be applied in a positive rather than negative manner. However, in practice, whether the present guidelines are improving therapy is yet to be established.

Risk assessment

5

5.1 How can risk be assessed?

Hypertension is a major risk factor for cardiovascular disease. However, in order to decide which patients to treat, and how, the risk for an individual patient must be assessed. This will allow the absolute benefit that patients can obtain from particular treatments to be weighed against the inconvenience/potential adverse effects of therapy. Major additional risk factors in addition to hypertension include age, sex, BMI, total cholesterol, LDL cholesterol, HDL cholesterol, fasting blood glucose, family history of premature cardiovascular disease, previous vascular events and smoking status.

5.2 What are the minimum data required for risk assessment?

Recently the American Heart Association and the American College of Cardiology endorsed the determination of global risk as measured by a multifactorial statistical model such as the Framingham Risk Score (Grundy *et al* 1999) (http://circ.ahajournals.org/cgi/content/full/100/13/1481). Well-established risk factors including age, sex, smoking history, blood pressure, total serum cholesterol, HDL cholesterol and blood glucose or history of diabetes are measured and entered into a risk calculation model, of which there are currently a number available (Greenland *et al* 2001). The assessment can be paper or computer based.

Modern risk-assessment tools are reasonably reliable and should be used more widely. However, many of the available risk-assessment models rely heavily on data from the Framingham study. As the Framingham study included few patients with diabetes in the original cohort, a number of risk-prediction programmes may thus underestimate the risk attributable to diabetes, and there is urgent need for an improved risk calculation equation applicable to this increasingly prevalent patient group. Furthermore, over the past few years a number of newer risk factors for coronary heart disease have emerged including homocysteine, C-reactive protein and lipoprotein (a). As yet, none of these factors has emerged as a convincing method of improving risk assessment. Finally, recent data from the Framingham Study have clearly demonstrated that pulse pressure (the difference between systolic and diastolic pressure) is the best predictor of coronary heart disease risk in patients over 50 years of age and most risk-assessment tools continue to be based on systolic and diastolic pressure.

5.3   Who is at particular risk?

A number of groups are at particular risk. They include subjects with known cardiovascular disease and those who have already suffered a cardiovascular event such as a myocardial infarction or stroke. In addition, patients with type 2 diabetes are also at increased risk (Haffner *et al* 1998) (*see Ch. 10*). Indeed, recent data demonstrate that subjects with type 2 diabetes are at the same risk as non-diabetic patients after myocardial infarction (*Fig. 5.1*). The exact reasons for this increased risk associated with type 2 diabetes remain unclear, but may relate in part to the clustering of other risk factors with this condition. In particular, as many as 80% of patients with type 2 diabetes will be hypertensive and the majority of patients with this condition will die from cardiovascular disease. However, even in the absence of other known risk factors, patients with diabetes remain at increased risk and type 2 diabetes can rightly be regarded as a vascular rather than an endocrine disorder.

5.4   What level of risk should be treated?

The BHS guidelines (Ramsay *et al* 1999) recommend that in addition to antihypertensive treatment, drug therapy to reduce cardiovascular risk should also be considered. Aspirin is recommended both for the secondary prevention of cardiovascular disease and also in subjects over the age of 50 whose blood pressure is controlled and who have a 10-year coronary heart disease risk of >15%. Statin therapy is recommended for subjects with hypertension and a total cholesterol of 5.0 mmol/l or greater and established vascular disease; or a 10-year coronary heart disease risk of ≥15%. The joint British guidelines state that even subjects whose 10-year risk of coronary heart disease is between 10–15% may be expected to benefit from blood pressure and cholesterol reduction.

5.5   Should absolute or relative risk be used?

Most guidelines recommend using an individual patient's absolute risk of a subsequent cardiovascular event when making the decision to institute therapeutic intervention. Such an approach has both advantages and disadvantages. Using the approach based on risk assessment, both the patient and the physician are provided with data that will specifically quantify the risk and the expected reduction in that risk following successful intervention. However, current guidelines are heavily reliant on risk-prediction equations such as those produced by the Framingham Study. Such equations cannot always be extrapolated to all patient populations. For example, there were very few patients with type 2 diabetes in the

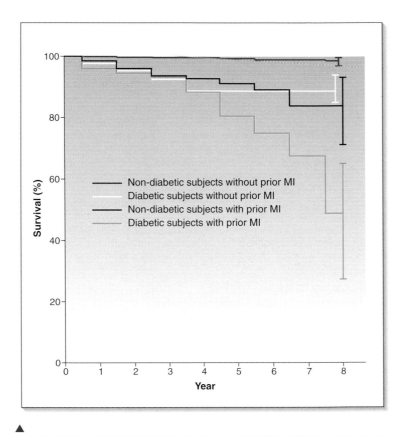

▲

Fig. 5.1 Diabetes and cardiovascular risk. Kaplan–Meier estimates of the probability of death from coronary heart disease in 1059 subjects with type 2 diabetes and 1378 non-diabetic subjects with and without prior myocardial infarction. MI, myocardial infarction. I bars indicate 95% confidence intervals. (From Haffner *et al* 1998, with permission. Copyright © 1998 Massachusetts Medical Society. All rights reserved.)

original Framingham cohort and thus risk-prediction equations based on Framingham may significantly underestimate the risk in type 2 diabetics. Recently, data from Framingham have shown that diastolic blood pressure predicts risk in patients under the age of 50 years, whilst in patients over 50, systolic and pulse pressure are better predictors of coronary heart disease. Finally, use of current evidence-based models of absolute risk will favour treatment of certain groups, for example the elderly rather than the young, men rather than women and smokers in favour of non-smokers. Whether in the future we treat on the basis of life years gained, or events prevented, is a debate that will have to be addressed by society as a whole.

5.6 What is an NNT?

The term 'NNT' stands for 'number needed to treat'. As suggested, this is simply the number of people who need to receive a particular treatment for one of them to achieve the desired benefit. The NNT for a particular intervention can be calculated simply as *1 divided by the absolute risk reduction observed for that therapy*. NNTs are a useful way of measuring benefit, or harm, from a particular trial, and comparing results (*see Tables 10.1 and 11.1* for examples). However, subject characteristics, duration of therapy and outcome measure are also important considerations when comparing NNTs.

 PATIENT QUESTIONS

5.7 Should I know my own risk of cardiovascular disease?

Not everyone wishes to know their risk for future cardiovascular disease. However, an increasing number of people do. Indeed, knowing one's own risk can be reassuring and/or help people take responsibility for appropriate lifestyle modification aimed at reducing risk. For those who are interested, a number of web sites provide risk calculators, for example:
http://www.hyp.ac.uk/bhs/managemt.html
http://www.medcal.mirai.co.uk/
http://www.mrfc2000fsnet.co.uk

5.8 How can I find out about the latest guidelines regarding hypertension and cardiovascular risk?

The best place to look for information about this is on the web. A number of excellent sites exist including:
http://www.hyp.ac.uk/bhs/managemt.html

Lifestyle intervention

6

BLOOD PRESSURE REDUCTION

6.1 Does salt restriction reduce blood pressure?

Consistent with an association between excess salt and raised blood pressure, dietary salt restriction results in a fall in blood pressure (Midgley *et al* 1996). In normotensives sodium restriction causes only a modest blood pressure reduction of ~1 mmHg systolic pressure drop per 100 mmol decrease in daily sodium intake. However, the reductions in hypertensive patients are much more substantial, achieving falls of ~6 systolic and 2 mmHg diastolic blood pressures per 100 mmol decrease in daily sodium intake. There is evidence that some patients are particularly sensitive to the effects of sodium on blood pressure. Salt-sensitive patients (≥10 mmHg systolic BP difference between low-salt and high-salt diets) have poorer prognosis than non-salt-sensitive patients (*Fig. 6.1*). Salt reduction is also an important adjunct to pharmacological blood pressure control (Erwteman *et al* 1984). Several studies have shown that the benefits of antihypertensive therapy are amplified by salt restriction. For example, during treatment with thiazide and beta-blockade, salt restriction could allow a further 3 mmHg reduction of systolic blood pressure to be attained.

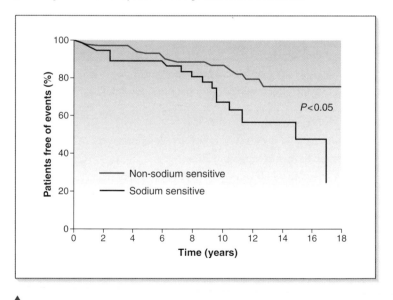

▲

Fig. 6.1 Salt sensitivity and mortality. Kaplan–Meier plots of total cardiovascular event-free survival on the basis of sodium sensitivity (≥10% BP difference on low- or high-sodium diets). (From Morimoto *et al* 1997, with permission of Elsevier Science.)

6.2　How can patients reduce their salt intake?

Patients should be given advice about dietary sources of sodium salt. It is most important that patients cut down on the amount, if any, of salt added after food preparation. Excessive use of salt for flavouring is habit forming, and although patients who are accustomed to using large amounts of excess salt may experience an initial loss of taste or flavour to food, this typically only lasts for a few weeks as they become re-acclimatized to a lower salt intake. Of greater concern may be the sodium content of food due to salt added during preparation stages. Patients should be given cautionary advice about foodstuffs with high salt content, particularly pre-prepared foods, and discouraged from adding excess salt during cooking. Foodstuffs that are low in salt should be encouraged, including fresh fruits and vegetables, and sodium salt substitutes, or other spices, e.g. lemon juice or pepper, may be used for taste, if necessary.

6.3　Does increased potassium intake reduce blood pressure?

The Rancho Bernardo project was a 12-year prospective cohort study that identified a strong inverse relationship between potassium intake and stroke risk, such that those in the lowest tertile of potassium ingestion had a relative risk of 2.6 in males and 4.8 in females, compared with the other tertiles (Khaw & Barrett-Connor 1987). This study suggested that each 10 mmol increase of dietary potassium intake was associated with a 40% reduction in the risk of stroke, which was independent of other dietary variables and known cardiovascular risk factors. The mechanisms of this apparent benefit are unclear, and several studies have examined the potential influence of potassium supplementation on blood pressure. One placebo-controlled study examined daily supplementation with potassium chloride, and found no effect on requirement for antihypertensive medication, the primary end-point of the study (Grimm et al 1990). Other large trials have found no reduction of blood pressure with similar dosages of potassium, while the results of several smaller studies have been mixed. At present, therefore, it appears that potassium supplementation is not effective in reducing blood pressure and is not recommended. However, no adverse effects of additional potassium intake have been identified, and it may provide a safe substitute for dietary sodium salt.

6.4　Is obesity linked with hypertension?

Obesity is defined as a body mass index greater than 30 kg/m^2 (Erwteman et al 1984) and has been reported to contribute to as many as two-thirds of cases of hypertension (Cassano et al 1990). In particular, waist:hip ratio serves as a measure of central 'abdominal' adiposity, which is more strongly linked to the risk of future hypertension, independent of body weight.

Moreover, obesity is linked to a variety of mechanisms that predispose to increased cardiovascular risk among hypertensive individuals, including activation of the sympathetic nervous system, dyslipidaemia, altered sodium handling, and insulin resistance. Therefore, obesity not only increases blood pressure, but also significantly enhances cardiovascular risk beyond that conferred by hypertension alone. In 1998, it was estimated that in England alone obesity imposed an additional healthcare burden of £457 million, predominantly through its effects on hypertension and cardiovascular disease risk. Follow-up in the Nurses' Health Study and the Health Professionals Follow-up Study over 18 and 10 years respectively showed that weight gain was significantly associated with increased risk of developing hypertension (*Fig. 6.2*).

6.5   What are the benefits of weight reduction?

Given the strong links between obesity and hypertension, it is hardly surprising that weight reduction offers an easily identifiable target in patient management. Several clinical trials, in both normotensive and hypertensive individuals, have demonstrated that loss of excess weight reduces both systolic and diastolic blood pressure to an extent proportional to total weight loss (Blumenthal *et al* 2000). Weight loss coupled to increased physical activity is additionally associated with increased basal metabolic rate, more efficient aerobic metabolism, increased insulin sensitivity, and improved general sense of well-being. Overall a fall of ~7/5 mmHg can be expected (Blumenthal *et al* 2000). Other benefits attributable to weight loss include improved lipid profile, normalization of vascular responsiveness and reduction in cardiac sympathetic drive, all of which serve to reduce overall cardiovascular risk. It is estimated that a 10% weight reduction in patients with an initial weight of 100 kg or over can lead to substantial benefits, outlined in Box 6.1. In practice, all hypertensive patients should have their weight measured, and those individuals with a BMI of 25 or more should be particularly encouraged to lose weight. The Treatment of Mild Hypertension Study provided evidence that the effectiveness of weight loss is additive to that achieved by antihypertensive medication.

BOX 6.1 Benefits of weight reduction (Royal College of Physicians of London 1998)

10% weight loss in those weighing 100 kg or more at baseline results in:

- substantial fall in systolic and diastolic blood pressure
- fall of 10% in total cholesterol
- greater than 50% reduction in the risk of developing diabetes
- a 30–40% fall in diabetes-related deaths
- a 20–25% fall in total mortality.

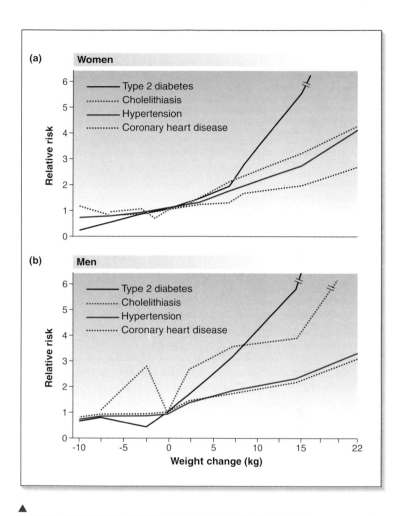

Fig. 6.2 Relation between the change in weight and relative risk of type 2 diabetes, hypertension, coronary heart disease, and cholelithiasis: **A.** for change of weight among women in the Nurses' Health Study, initially 30–55 years of age, who were followed for up to 18 years; **B.** for change of weight among men in the Health Professionals Follow-up Study, initially 40–65 years of age, who were followed for up to 10 years. (From Willet *et al* 1999, with permission. Copyright © 1999 Massachusetts Medical Society. All rights reserved.)

6.6 How can weight loss be achieved?

Just as obesity itself results from the interaction of several factors, its treatment requires a multifold approach directed at changing and maintaining lifestyle. Dietary advice should address total calorific intake, and aim to reduce the proportion of diet made up of highly refined carbohydrates. The goals of weight loss and an ideal target weight should be established with the patient at the outset of a weight loss programme. Depending on the severity of obesity and the degree of patient motivation a number of different methods are available. Most involve a multifactorial approach involving nutritional education, encouragement to moderate alcohol intake, and programmes to promote increased physical activity. Unfortunately, the results of lifestyle modification can be poor, with most trials demonstrating a return to baseline weight within a few years for many patients. Drug therapy may be appropriate for carefully selected and motivated patients, although the long-term usefulness of this approach has not yet been tested. Two of the most promising anti-obesity drugs at present are sibutramine and orlistat, which appear to be very effective at achieving and possibly maintaining reduced weight. Since patients receiving these drugs require careful selection and close monitoring, they remain largely confined to specialist clinics, and are not suitable for more widespread use.

6.7 Is drinking alcohol associated with an increased blood pressure?

There are extensive observational data linking excess alcohol consumption with hypertension (*see Q. 2.13*). The majority of data indicate a positive, linear association between the level of alcohol intake and blood pressure in men and women. Moreover, high levels of alcohol intake are associated with increased risk of developing hypertension, both across and within populations. In a recent Canadian study, excess alcohol consumption was thought to be a major attributable cause of hypertension in up to 4% of cases among males aged 60–64 years. Whilst these studies do not prove cause and effect, a causal or contributory relationship is very likely, given the consistency of substantial observational data that has accrued. Furthermore, the pattern of consumption appears to be important; binge drinking appears to be associated with increased risk, even after adjusting for total consumption (*Fig. 6.3*).

6.8 Does reducing alcohol intake lower blood pressure?

Several large randomized controlled clinical trials have examined the effect of reducing alcohol consumption on blood pressure amongst hypertensive individuals. Interventions with advice to reduce alcohol, abstain from

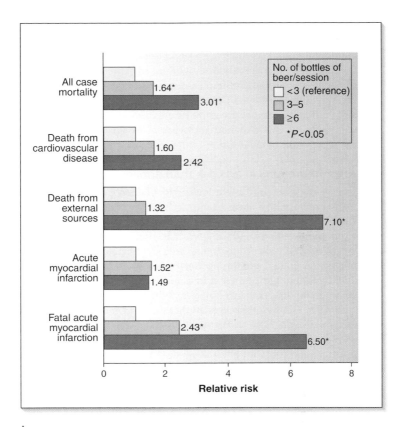

Fig. 6.3 Relative risk of mortality and major morbidity associated with drinking pattern (number of drinks/session). Data from the Finnish prospective population study are adjusted for age and overall alcohol consumption. (From: Kauhanen *et al* 1997, with permission of the BMJ Publishing Group.)

alcohol, and cognitive behavioural therapy have all been examined, and the majority demonstrate a 5–8 mmHg reduction in systolic and 2–3 mmHg reduction in diastolic blood pressures. However, these studies are likely to underestimate the potential benefits of alcohol moderation on blood pressure for several reasons. In many of the trials, alcohol consumption often fell substantially in the control and intervention groups, minimizing the apparent benefit and, furthermore, patients may not have adhered to the alcohol-reducing interventions, as the majority of studies depended on patient reporting for data collection with no objective assessment of compliance. Observations from uncontrolled interventions provide consistent evidence of a fall in blood pressure associated with alcohol moderation. Patients should be encouraged to reduce overall alcohol consumption, and certainly at least to a level that conforms with more widely applicable suggested alcohol limits. In particular, binge drinking should be discouraged as this is associated with rapid rises in blood pressure, and appears to be most closely linked to overall cardiovascular risk. It should be emphasized that excess alcohol consumption will antagonize the effects of most antihypertensive agents, and abstinence will, therefore, make blood pressure control easier to attain.

6.9 Are non-drinkers at less risk than drinkers?

Non-drinkers are probably at lowest risk of developing or aggravating hypertension, with a linear relation between increasing consumption and rising blood pressure. However, consideration of the relationship between alcohol consumption and cardiovascular risk, or total mortality, is more complicated. A J-shaped curve has been identified in many observational population studies, and this has been subjected to several interpretations. Some have interpreted these data as indicating that moderate alcohol consumption may be beneficial, and perhaps more desirable than complete abstinence. Others have suggested that the abstinent group may include many who are at high cardiovascular risk and who take no alcohol because of a specific contraindication or concurrent illness. Furthermore, the Copenhagen City Heart Study suggested that wine drinking may be less harmful than beer or spirit drinking, although this may be associated with different patterns of consumption and other lifestyle factors (*Fig. 6.4*). The debate remains open, and the pragmatic approach might be to suggest that patients moderate alcohol intake to as close to abstinence as possible; certainly, non-drinkers should not be encouraged to consume alcohol.

6.10 Does exercise reduce blood pressure?

Acute physical exercise is associated with a short-lived rise in systemic blood pressure, but perhaps somewhat paradoxically, there is now compelling evidence that regular exercise can make a substantial contribution to the treatment of mild hypertension (Higashi *et al* 1999). This reduction in blood pressure (~8/4 mmHg) appears to be greatest among those with lowest levels of physical activity at baseline, and correlates less well with the increase in maximal exercise capacity. In other words, the greatest benefits can be achieved by a modest improvement in the level of physical activity among the most sedentary patients. Clinical trials have shown that in patients with moderate to severe hypertension, a 16-week programme of regular aerobic exercise led not only to a significant reduction in blood pressure, but also to a reduction in left ventricular mass

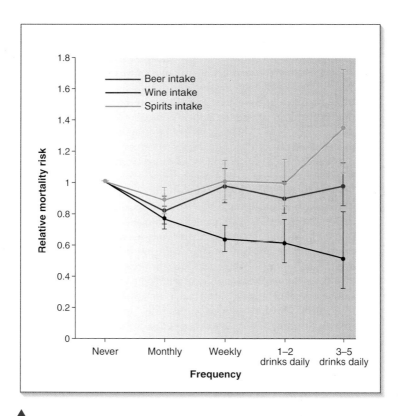

Fig. 6.4 Relative mortality risk associated with frequency of alcohol consumption, for beer, wine, and spirit intake. Data from the Copenhagen City Heart Study. (From: Gronbaek *et al* 1995, with permission of the BMJ Publishing Group.)

index. Moreover, several studies have shown that the effects of exercise on blood pressure are independent of, and in addition to, any change in body mass index that may accompany increased activity as part of a global lifestyle modification approach. The risks of regular moderate exercise are small. In predisposed individuals, exercise may precipitate asthma attacks, and vigorous exercise can lead to angina, and rarely myocardial infarction. It should be noted that even in patients with established atherosclerotic disease, with or without raised blood pressure, regular exercise is advocated to reduce the risk of cardiovascular death. Therefore, in hypertensive patients the small potential increase in short-term risk should not be considered an important limitation, as it is vastly offset by the benefits of taking regular exercise.

6.11 What type of exercise is best?

Most of the studies of the effects of exercise on blood pressure have examined dynamic exercise, rather than resistive exercise. Therefore, walking, cycling and non-competitive swimming are to be encouraged, and dynamic exercise of moderate intensity for 45–60 minutes, three to four time per week, appears to be at least as effective at lowering blood pressure as vigorous exercise. There appears to be no additional benefit from following a daily regimen, and the antihypertensive effects are less pronounced when shorter exercise durations (e.g. 20–30 minutes) are used.

6.12 Is relaxation therapy effective?

There has been considerable interest in the relationships between perceived stress and the development of hypertension and cardiovascular disease risk. Certainly, situational stress can cause short-lived increases in blood pressure, among otherwise normotensive individuals. Classical 'white-coat effect' is one example of this, although the degree to which this pattern of blood pressure responsiveness may predispose to the development of sustained high blood pressure remains somewhat unclear. A recent study has shown that the rise in blood pressure due to performing a stressful cognitive task is a strong predictor of progression of carotid atherosclerosis. At present, there is no evidence that stress management can prevent the development of hypertension. Among hypertensives, meta-analyses of single modality interventions to reduce stress (e.g. meditation, relaxation therapy, problem-solving skill development) suggest that there is no significant improvement in blood pressure. However, use of combined relaxation therapies has been shown to cause some improvement in blood pressure, which appears to be sustained beyond the treatment period. For example, a meta-analysis of individualized cognitive stress management using multiple approaches has found mean blood pressure reductions of 15/9 mmHg. Nevertheless, data from properly controlled randomized studies are still required to substantiate this result. In all hypertensive patients, the potential contribution of stress should be considered, and where it is felt to be important, stress management should be considered. The benefits of this are likely to be greater where treatment is tailored to the individual patient's needs, and where several modalities are combined.

CARDIOVASCULAR RISK REDUCTION

6.13 What other lifestyle factors are important?

Smoking is a potent risk factor for cardiovascular disease and half of all smokers die before reaching retirement age. Thus, smoking cessation is an important goal in all patients, especially those with hypertension. Indeed, a number of studies have shown that the risk of stroke decreases on stopping smoking although there is a variation in the estimate of how long it takes for risk to return to that of a non-smoker (2–10 years).

6.14 Is anything effective in helping patients stop smoking?

Both nicotine replacement and amfebutamone ('Zyban') are moderately effective in increasing the success rate of smoking cessation programmes. Both are available in the UK for suitable patients.

 PATIENT QUESTIONS

6.15 Can changing my lifestyle lower my blood pressure?

Certainly some lifestyle changes lead to a fall in blood pressure. Weight reduction in obese subjects has been shown to reduce blood pressure, as does reducing salt and alcohol intake. However, the expected effects are relatively modest and are likely only to be sufficient to normalize blood pressure in those with borderline hypertension. Nevertheless, they are important and everyone should attempt them in addition to undertaking more general lifestyle changes such as stopping smoking, eating five servings of fruit and vegetables per day, and taking more exercise.

6.16 Should I avoid exercise and stress?

There is no hard evidence that stress reduction leads to a fall in blood pressure. However, some individuals find relaxation exercises helpful. Gentle exercise should be encouraged in all patients, but it is not wise to undertake particularly strenuous exercise without first consulting your doctor, and first having good blood pressure control.

6.17 Do I need to be off work with my high blood pressure?

In almost all cases the answer is no. Very rarely people may be advised to rest at home, pregnant women for example, or even admitted to hospital, and for one or two professions you are not permitted to work until blood pressure control is achieved (e.g. airline pilots). However, in most cases hypertension does not require time off work.

PQ PATIENT QUESTIONS

Drug treatment for primary hypertension

7

PRACTICAL PRESCRIBING IN HYPERTENSION

7.1 Which drugs should be used first-line?

A number of factors will influence which drug is selected as first-line therapy for hypertension; including efficacy, side-effect profile and cost. Assuming that there are no contraindications to any of the main agents then most physicians would suggest that a β-blocker or thiazide diuretic should be used first-line. Indeed, these two agents have the most long-term follow-up data, are generally well tolerated and are relatively inexpensive. Interestingly, recent evidence suggest that β-blockers may be preferable in younger subjects, because of a higher response rate (Dickerson *et al* 1999). However, there seems to be little difference between the four main classes of antihypertensive drugs with regard to outcome measures including total and cardiovascular mortality (Neal *et al* 2000, Staessen *et al* 2001).

Similarly, in the elderly the STOP-2 (Hansson *et al* 1999a) trial found no evidence to suggest any difference between older (β-blockers and thiazides) and newer (calcium-channel blockers and angiotensin-converting enzyme (ACE) inhibitors) drugs (*see Table 11.2*). Nevertheless, at least one meta-analysis suggests that β-blockers may be less efficacious than diuretics in those with isolated systolic hypertension (Messerli *et al* 1998), and thus thiazide diuretics remain the first-choice of many in the elderly.

7.2 What is an appropriate interval before assessing the response to therapy?

Most antihypertensive drugs have their maximum blood pressure-lowering effect after 2–4 weeks, although thiazide diuretics may take slightly longer. Therefore, most physicians would suggest waiting for around 6 weeks before assessing the response to therapy. Moreover, if possible, blood pressure should be assessed on two separate occasions before making any therapeutic decisions. Nevertheless, in subjects with malignant hypertension or significant comorbidity it may be necessary to significantly shorten the review interval.

7.3 Should treatment be cumulative or rotational?

Opinions vary as to whether an additional drug should be prescribed if the first-line therapy fails to reduce blood pressure significantly or whether the initial drug should be substituted with another. Practically, if the initial blood pressure is only modestly elevated and target pressure is likely to be achieved with a single agent, then it makes sense to try another agent as monotherapy. Having said this, there is little point in making a substitution within a class; indeed the evidence suggests that there is a considerable relationship between the response to β-blockers and ACE inhibitors, and between thiazides and calcium-channel blockers (Dickerson *et al* 1999). Thus, if a patient fails to reach target on a β-blocker it would seem more sensible to try either a thiazide or calcium-channel blocker, and vice versa, since ACE inhibitors are likely to be no better than the original β-blocker.

Conversely, if the initial blood pressure is markedly elevated and the original drug produces a reasonable reduction in blood pressure (~10/5 mmHg), then it is probably wise to add-in another agent (*see Q. 7.4*).

7.4 Which drug combinations are effective?

The ABCD rule can be used to guide effective combination therapy (*see Box 7.1*). The aim is to use drugs in a synergistic manner where possible (*Fig. 7.1*). This usually involves selecting agents with different mechanisms of action: ACE inhibitors and β-blockers both inhibit the renin–angiotensin system, whereas thiazides and calcium-channel blockers are mainly vasodilators and actually activate the renin–angiotensin system. However, as many studies have recently shown, in order to reach targets, approximately two-thirds of patients are likely to require more than one antihypertensive drug.

BOX 7.1 Combination therapy

Step 1	Establish monotherapy
Step 2	**A** or **B** + **C** or **D**
Step 3	Add/substitute an α-blocker
Step 4	Reconsider secondary hypertension/specialist referral

A = Angiotensin-converting enzyme inhibitors
B = β-blockers
C = Calcium-channel blockers
D = Thiazide diuretics

7.5 Who should be referred for further investigation and management?

The main groups of patients who require specialist referral are given in Box 7.2. However, at what stage patients are referred will depend on a number of factors including established practice and local interests.

7.6 Are fixed-dose combinations useful?

Traditionally fixed-dose drug combinations have been frowned upon in the UK because of concerns over cost and the optimal dose combinations.

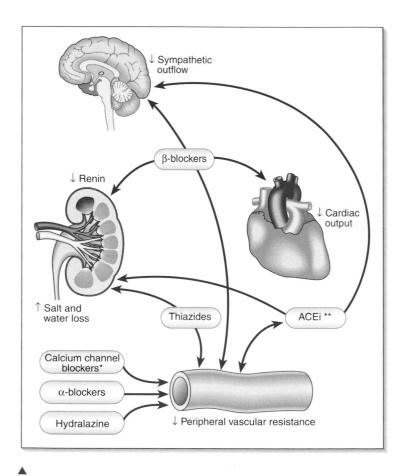

▲

Fig. 7.1 Sites of action of the main antihypertensive drugs.* Non-dihydropyridines also reduce cardiac output. ** ACEi, angiotensin-converting enzyme inhibitors. These drugs inhibit angiotensin II formation, which leads to vasodilatation, reduced aldosterone production, a fall in sympathetic activity and also reversal of cardiovascular remodelling.

Fortunately many of these issues have now been resolved and a number of fixed-dose combinations are currently available in the UK, e.g. co-amilozide, and Zestoretic (lisinopril and hydrochlorothiazide). These can be of considerable use in patients requiring polypharmacy – reducing the number of tablets patients are required to take each day and thus possibly improving compliance.

BOX 7.2 Suggested indications for specialist referral

- Hypertensive emergency (e.g. encephalopathy)
- Malignant or accelerated hypertension
- Hypertension at a young age (<20 years)
- Systolic hypertension in youth (<30 years)
- Suspected secondary hypertension
- Renal impairment
- Resistant hypertension (e.g. not at target on three drugs)
- Multiple drug intolerance
- Pregnancy
- 'Labile' blood pressure
- Suspected 'white-coat hypertension'

7.7 Is 24-hour control of blood pressure important?

The heart, brain and vasculature are exposed to cyclical changes in blood pressure continuously. Therefore, 24-hour control of blood pressure should be considered optimal. Indeed, there is evidence that left ventricular hypertrophy regresses more effectively with 24-hour blood pressure control. Thus, this should be the aim for all patients, and can be aided by using once-a-day drug preparations and avoiding drugs with short half-lives, such as standard-release nifedipine.

THIAZIDE DIURETICS

7.8 How do thiazides lower blood pressure?

Thiazide diuretics have been extensively used in the treatment of hypertension since the introduction of chlorothiazide in 1957. Thiazides are actively transported into collecting tubules in the kidney and inhibit the Na^+/Cl^- cotransporter in the distal convoluted tubule (*Fig. 7.2*). This results in increased sodium and water loss and, by virtue of increased sodium delivery to the distal nephron, a concomitant increase in potassium excretion.

The initial reduction in blood pressure observed with thiazides is accompanied by a ~15% reduction in extracellular volume, a fall in cardiac output and compensatory rise in peripheral vascular resistance. However, with chronic therapy the system 're-sets' because of counter-regulatory mechanisms, and cardiac output and peripheral vascular resistance return to normal but blood pressure remains lowered. Whether, volume depletion persists in this state is controversial but any reduction is certainly far less

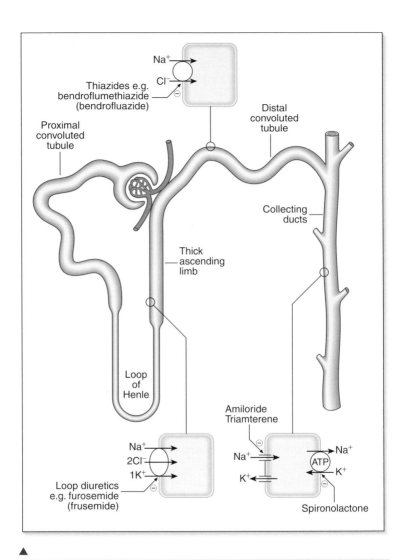

▲

Fig. 7.2 Sites of action of the main diuretics.

than that observed acutely. This has led to the suggestion that thiazide diuretics have other antihypertensive mechanisms. Indeed, vasodilatation in response to thiazides has been reported, but this is not thought to be due to inhibition of a vascular Na^+/Cl^- cotransporter.

7.9   What are the indications for their use?

There are no specific indications for the use of thiazide diuretics, but many suggest them as first-line therapy for the majority of patients, especially in the elderly.

7.10   What are the contraindications to their use?

The main contraindication is gout, and a more complete list is given in Box 7.3. It should also be noted that thiazides are ineffective in reducing blood pressure in patients with renal impairment (serum creatinine >150 μmol/l), and their antihypertensive effect is markedly reduced by concomitant administration of non-steroidal anti-inflammatory drugs (NSAIDs).

BOX 7.3   Contraindications to thiazide diuretics

■ Gout
■ Refractory hypokalaemia or hyponatraemia
■ Renal impairment
■ Severe hepatic impairment
■ Avoid in pregnancy

7.11   What are the adverse effects of thiazides?

Thiazide diuretics have few side-effects when used in low doses to treat hypertension. The main side-effects are gout, impotence (<2%), hypokalaemia and hyponatraemia, postural hypotension, and photosensitive rashes. At low dosage (e.g. 2.5 mg bendroflumethiazide (bendrofluazide)) any tendency to hyperglycaemia and dyslipidaemia is *not* clinically significant.

7.12   What is the evidence-base for thiazides?

Repeated studies have demonstrated the efficacy of thiazide diuretics in hypertensive subjects (Neal *et al* 2000, Staessen *et al* 2001) (*Fig. 7.3*). Indeed, they probably have more evidence for their use than any other class of antihypertensive drug, and certainly the greatest safety data.

7.13   What factors influence their efficacy?

Thiazide diuretics are more effective in patients with low plasma renin activity, such as the elderly and black subjects. They are slightly less effective in younger subjects because younger people often have high renin levels. However, they are markedly less effective in patients with renal impairment (serum creatinine >150 μmol/l), and those subjects taking non-steroidal anti-inflammatory drugs.

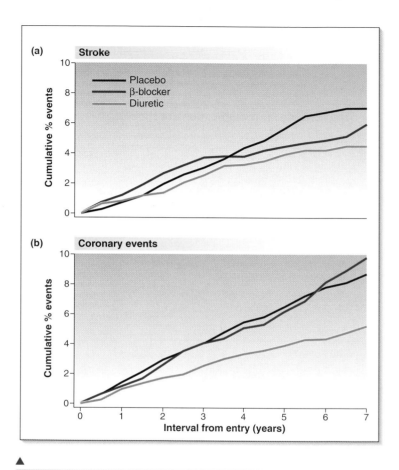

Fig. 7.3 Results of the MRC trial in hypertensive older adults. Effect of thiazide, β-blocker and placebo on stroke (**A**) and coronary events (**B**) in the MRC trial of treatment of hypertension in older adults. After adjustment for other confounding variables only the thiazide significantly reduced both events. (From MRC Working Party 1992, with permission of the BMJ Publishing Group.)

7.14 Is there a dose relationship?

Thiazide diuretics do not exhibit a dose relationship. Many of the original trials were conducted with relatively high doses of drugs, but subsequent studies have demonstrated that increasing the dose does not lead to a greater blood pressure reduction, just more side-effects. Therefore, 2.5 or even 1.25 mg of bendroflumethiazide (bendrofluazide) should be the standard antihypertensive dose.

7.15   Are there differences between drugs?

No. There are no clinically significant differences between drugs.

β-BLOCKERS

7.16   How do β-blockers lower blood pressure?

Chronic therapy with β-blockers lower blood pressure in four main ways:

- reduced cardiac output
- inhibition of the renin–angiotensin system by reducing renin secretion
- reduced sympathetic nervous system activity
- baroreceptor 'resetting' and reduced baroreceptor sensitivity.

However, most of the acute effect of β-blockade is due to reduced cardiac output, rather than peripheral vasodilatation. Indeed, vascular β-adrenoceptors cause peripheral vasodilatation; thus β-blockers – particularly non-selective agents – initially increase peripheral vascular resistance, which returns to normal with continued therapy.

7.17   What are the indications for their use?

In patients with hypertension and angina, β-blockers are indicated unless there are strong contraindications to their use, such as coexisting asthma, chronic obstructive pulmonary disease or heart failure. Indeed, in the MRC Hypertension Trial β-blockers were most effective in preventing myocardial infarction in non-smokers. There is also strong evidence to support the use of β-blockade in hypertensive patients who have suffered a myocardial infarction as these agents reduce sudden death, decrease re-infarction rates, and increase life expectancy (Freemantle *et al* 1999). The incidence of hypertension in patients with type 2 diabetes is high – between 70 and 80%, depending on the definition of high blood pressure used. The results of the UKPDS showed that in patients with type 2 diabetes, blood pressure reduction with the β-blocker atenolol was equally effective as the ACE inhibitor captopril in reducing the incidence of stroke. However, neither drug significantly decreased the incidence of myocardial infarction. A number of large randomized, controlled studies have demonstrated that β-blockade is beneficial in patients with heart failure, but it needs to be introduced with care.

7.18   What are the contraindications to their use?

 Compelling contraindications to the use of β-blockade include asthma and chronic obstructive pulmonary disease. It should also be noted that if given inappropriately without adequate follow-up or supervision, β-blockers can worsen heart failure and should currently, therefore, be prescribed to treat heart failure by hospital specialists or specialist heart failure nurses. Although traditionally β-blockers have been avoided in patients with peripheral vascular disease (PVD), such patients commonly have angina and are at increased risk of myocardial infarction and, therefore, probably stand to benefit substantially from β-blocker therapy. Indeed, pooled analyses of trials in patients with PVD demonstrated no significant deterioration in claudication in patients taking β-blockers. Nevertheless, one may choose to use a highly selective β_1-adrenergic blocker in such patients. Finally, in patients with heart block β-blockers are absolutely contraindicated.

7.19 What are their adverse effects?

 In general, β-blockers are well tolerated by most patients. However, some individuals develop annoying side-effects, especially if treated with high doses of these agents. Central effects of β-blockade include tiredness and fatigue, nightmares, insomnia or vivid dreams. Such side-effects are less common with less lipid-soluble agents such as atenolol. A number of small studies have also suggested that depression is associated with β-blockade. A meta-analysis (Patten 1990) showed no difference in the prevalence of depression when β-blockers were compared to other antihypertensive agents. Sexual dysfunction is also a side-effect of β-blockade. However, in the MRC blood pressure trial, thiazide diuretics produced a similar level of sexual dysfunction, which was possibly dose related. Recent data from the TOHMS study (Grimm *et al* 1997) reported a higher incidence of erectile dysfunction in men taking diuretics rather than the other major classes of antihypertensives.

7.20 What is the evidence-base for these drugs?

The evidence for the use of β-blockers as first-line treatment for hypertension is a strong one. The majority of the early randomized placebo-controlled trials including the MRC and HAPPY study used β-blockers and diuretics. More recently, two large studies have compared antihypertensive regimes based on β-blockade or diuretics against newer agents including ACE inhibitors and calcium-channel blockers (STOP-2 trial) and against ACE inhibitors (CAPP study). STOP-2 failed to find any meaningful differences between older and newer drugs; and in the CAPP study there were more actual strokes in the ACE inhibitor-treated group than in the diuretic or β-blocker group. The evidence-base for the use of β-blockers in the treatment of isolated systolic hypertension is less strong and the weight of evidence would favour diuretic therapy over β-blockade in this increasingly prevalent patient group.

7.21 What factors influence their efficacy?

Data from a large number of studies suggest that β-blockers are especially effective in young Caucasian patients and less effective in black Afro-Caribbean subjects. This may be due in part to the fact that β-blockers act to decrease renin release from the kidney and black subjects are more likely to have volume-expanded low renin hypertension, as indeed are older subjects. In addition, there are differences in the frequency of certain β_2-adrenoceptor polymorphisms between black and white subjects, which may also influence responses to β-blockade. It is also true that β-blockers are especially effective in patients with a resting tachycardia.

7.22 Are there differences between drugs in this class?

There are a number of important differences between β-blockers. At a basic level β-blockers can be classified according to their cardioselectivity. Cardioselectivity (i.e. β_1 selectivity) theoretically limits the potentially adverse effect of β_2-blockade on pulmonary function and peripheral vascular resistance. Drugs such as atenolol, acebutolol, metoprolol and nebivolol exhibit a relatively high degree of β_1 selectivity. In addition, nebivolol promotes peripheral vasodilatation via release of nitric oxide. β-blockers also vary in their degree of lipid-solubility: agents that are lipid-soluble such as propranolol and metoprolol will cross the blood–brain barrier and produce more central nervous system effects, e.g. nightmares. In addition, they also tend to have a shorter duration of action since they are inactivated more rapidly in the liver. Atenolol is an example of a less lipid-soluble β-blocker.

CALCIUM-CHANNEL BLOCKERS

7.23 What is their mechanism of action?

There are two main types of calcium-channel blockers (*see Table 7.1*). All calcium-channel blockers act to inhibit calcium influx into muscle cells by blocking L-type calcium channels. The dihydropyridines lower blood pressure by reducing peripheral vascular tone and contractility, which leads to vasodilatation and a fall in peripheral vascular resistance. Usually this is

TABLE 7.1 Classes of calcium-channel blockers

	Dihydropyridines	Non-dihydropyridines
Examples	Nifedipine, amlodipine, lercanidipine	Verapamil, diltiazem
Effect on heart rate	Increase	Decrease
Site of action	Vasculature	Vasculature and heart
Side-effects	Headache, ankle swelling Flushing	Constipation, heart failure Heart block

accompanied by a reflex increase in heart rate and sympathetic activation, which is why a combination therapy with a β-blocker is often used. The non-dihydropyridines also cause a fall in peripheral vascular resistance but in addition reduce myocardial contractility and heart rate. This leads to a fall in cardiac output, which contributes to their blood pressure-lowering effects. In contrast to the dihydropyridines, there tends to be no reflex rise in heart rate with these drugs.

7.24 What are the indications for their use?

One of the most compelling indications for the use of calcium-channel blockers is isolated systolic hypertension in the elderly (*see Qs 11.6–11.17*). Of three placebo-controlled trials in this patient group, two – SystEur (nitrendipine) and SystChina (nitrendipine) – used a long-acting calcium-channel blocker. Patients with hypertension and coexisting angina may also potentially benefit from a calcium-channel blocker, either a dihydropyridine or a non-dihydropyridine. However, a meta-analysis based on 16 trials using nifedipine in patients with chronic angina suggested an increase in cardiac event rates. Therefore, short-acting calcium-channel blockers cannot be recommended in this patient group (Furberg *et al* 1995), and are probably best avoided in general. Nevertheless, two large studies have confirmed the efficacy and safety of long-acting dihydropyridines (nifedipine LA – Brown *et al* 2000) and non-dihydropyridines (diltiazem – Hansson *et al* 2000) in hypertensive patients, as have meta-analyses.

A large number of randomized trials have demonstrated that antihypertensive therapy reduces morbidity and mortality from cardiovascular disease in subjects with diabetes. Indeed, since diabetic subjects are at higher risk, the absolute risk reduction with antihypertensive therapy is greater than in non-diabetics. Low-dose thiazide diuretics, β-blockers and ACE inhibitors have all proven to be effective antihypertensive agents in individuals with diabetes. However, in recent studies comparing hypertensive subjects with diabetes randomized to an ACE inhibitor or calcium-channel blocker there were fewer coronary heart disease events in the ACE inhibitor group (Estacio *et al* 1998, Tatti *et al* 1998). However, recent data from the SystEur study, which was based on the calcium-channel blocker, nitrendipine, showed a greater benefit in the diabetic subjects randomized to nitrendipine than in non-diabetic subjects. Therefore, calcium-channel blockers probably should not be used first-line in diabetics, except in the elderly, but may be useful add-on drugs.

7.25 What are the contraindications to their use?

HEART FAILURE

Since many calcium-channel blockers are negatively inotropic, the use of these agents in patients with heart failure has been a matter of much speculation. A number of trials have examined the effect of calcium-channel blockers in individuals with left ventricular dysfunction. In one study the calcium-channel blocker amlodipine was added in for patients already taking diuretics and ACE inhibitors. No difference was observed in overall survival between the subjects taking amlodipine and those who received placebo (Packer *et al* 1996). Smaller placebo-controlled studies have also failed to demonstrate differences in clinical outcomes in patients with heart failure treated with either diltiazem or felodipine. Thus calcium-channel blockers are probably safe in heart failure, but should be introduced cautiously. However, non-dihydropyridines are probably best avoided.

OTHER CONTRAINDICATIONS

The non-dihydropyridine calcium-channel blocker, verapamil, produces partial blockade of both the AV and SA nodes in addition to a negative inotropic effect and, therefore, should not be used in combination with β-blockade. Calcium-channel blockers should also be used with caution in patients with aortic stenosis and heart block.

7.26 What are their adverse effects?

Adverse effects attributable to calcium-channel blockers will vary according to the type of agent used (*see Table 7.1*). Side-effects associated with the dihydropyridine class of calcium-channel blockers include flushing, headaches, postural dizziness, palpitations and tachycardia and ankle oedema. These side-effects are all relatively more common with shorter-acting preparations, and in women. Ankle oedema is especially troublesome and results from leakage of fluid from the capillary bed because of vasodilatation, and usually resolves with bed rest or dose reduction. The non-dihydropyridines especially, can worsen heart failure, and precipitate heart block in some patients.

7.27 What is the evidence-base for their use?

Until recently the evidence-base for the use of calcium-channel blockers was small. However, two recent large studies, INSIGHT (*Fig. 7.4*) using nifedipine GITS (Brown *et al* 2000), and NORDIL using diltiazem (Hansson *et al* 2000), both demonstrated that calcium-channel blockade was equally effective at reducing cardiovascular events as regimes based on diuretics or β-blockers. Furthermore, meta-analysis of the cardiovascular protection produced by blood pressure reduction based on nine randomized trials involving 62 605 hypertensive patients concluded that it is blood pressure reduction *per se* that produces most benefit and all antihypertensive agents had similar long-term efficacy and safety. However, the authors concluded that calcium-channel blockers might be especially effective in preventing stroke (Staessen *et al* 2001).

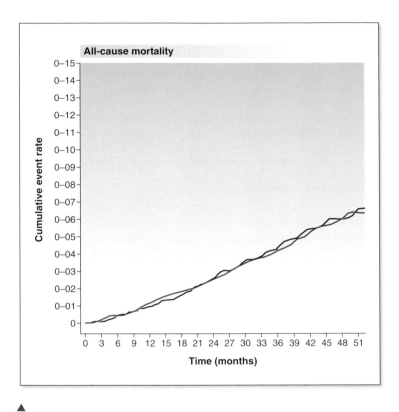

▲

Fig. 7.4 Results of the INSIGHT Study. Effect of nifedipine (black line) and co-amilozide (red line) on total mortality amongst hypertensive patients. There was no difference between agents (*P* = 0.95). (From Brown *et al* 2000, with permission of Elsevier Science.)

7.28 What factors influence their efficacy?

Calcium-channel blockers appear to be equally effective as other classes of drugs in reducing blood pressure. In particular, calcium-channel blockers are as effective as diuretics in the elderly, and in black African patients may be more effective than β-blockers or ACE inhibitors.

ANGIOTENSIN-CONVERTING ENZYME (ACE) INHIBITORS

7.29 What are their mechanisms of action?

Angiotensin-converting enzyme (ACE) inhibitors act by inhibiting the conversion of angiotensin I, a largely inactive decapeptide, to the potent

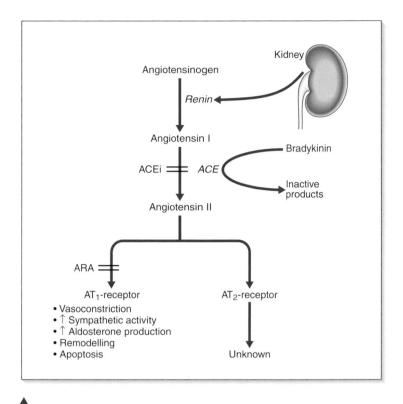

Fig. 7.5 The renin–angiotensin system and sites of drug action. Renin is released from the macula densa in the kidney and catalyses the formation of angiotensin I from angiotensinogen (which is made in the liver). Circulating and bound angiotensin-converting enzyme (ACE) then catalyses the formation of angiotensin II, which acts on two distinct receptors: AT_1 and AT_2. ACE also catalyses the breakdown of bradykinin, which is a potent vasodilator. Angiotensin-converting enzyme inhibitors (ACEi) thus probably reduce blood pressure by inhibiting angiotensin II formation and increasing bradykinin levels. AT_1 receptors are responsible for most of the known actions of angiotensin II, and are blocked by angiotensin-receptor antagonists (ARA).

vasoconstrictor peptide angiotensin II (*Fig. 7.5*). The observation that these drugs are effective antihypertensive agents, despite the fact that the majority of patients with essential hypertension have low or normal renin levels, suggested further mechanisms of action. Indeed, since ACE also degrades the vasodilator peptide bradykinin, ACE inhibitors will also produce vasodilatation by potentiating the levels of this peptide. This has recently been proved, since administration of a bradykinin receptor blocker HOE-140 has been shown to blunt the hypotensive effect of ACE inhibition by approximately 20%. In addition to direct vasoconstriction, angiotensin II increases noradrenaline (norepinephrine) release presynaptically, and thus ACE inhibitors will also decrease sympathetic activation. Finally, as bradykinin enhances the synthesis of a number of vasodilator prostaglandins, ACE inhibition will increase circulating levels of these compounds, leading to further vasodilatation.

7.30 What are the indications for their use?

There are a number of compelling indications for the use of ACE inhibitors. A high percentage of patients with hypertension have coexisting heart failure. Indeed, as many as a third to a half of patients in some of the heart failure studies have been hypertensive. The greatest benefits from ACE inhibition occur in patients with ejection fractions <25% and are noticeable within 3 months of initiating therapy.

The presence of type 1 diabetes is another compelling indication for the use of ACE inhibition. Independently of their blood pressure-lowering effect, ACE inhibitors slow the progression of renal damage in subjects with microalbuminuria or proteinuria. Therefore, they may be considered to be first-line therapy for type 1 diabetics. Interestingly, ACE inhibitors may also reduce the progression of renal disease in patients with type 2 diabetes, and recent evidence suggest that they may also retard the development of diabetes. Finally, subjects with any form of chronic renal disease may also derive benefit from treatment with ACE inhibitors, with the strong proviso that renal artery stenosis has been excluded as a cause of the chronic renal disease, and that they are used with close supervision.

7.31 What are the contraindications to their use?

 ACE inhibitors should be used with caution in subjects with peripheral vascular disease (PVD) because of the significant association between PVD and renal artery stenosis. Indeed, renal artery stenosis is a contraindication to the use of ACE inhibitors, as it may precipitate acute renal failure (*see Qs 9.19–9.30*). Therefore, it is important to monitor urea and electrolytes in all subjects around 10 days after initiating therapy with an ACE inhibitor.

Subjects taking high doses of diuretics (thus activating the renin–angiotensin system) are at increased risk of first-dose hypotension following ACE inhibition and it is often advisable to decrease the diuretic dosage when starting such subjects on an ACE inhibitor. If this is not possible, institute ACE inhibitor therapy under close medical supervision. In addition, since renal function is also regulated by prostaglandins, subjects on chronic therapy with non-steroidal anti-inflammatory drugs are also at increased risk of renal failure when started on ACE inhibition, especially if there is underlying renal disease. Moreover, NSAIDs blunt the blood pressure-lowering effect of ACE inhibitors.

Finally, ACE inhibition is absolutely contraindicated in pregnancy, and women of childbearing age should not be started on ACE inhibition unless they are established on adequate contraception. Indeed, ACE inhibitors are associated with pulmonary hypoplasia, fetal skull hypoplasia, growth retardation and fetal renal failure when used in the second and third trimesters (Briggs 1998).

7.32   What are their adverse effects?

 The major adverse effect associated with ACE inhibition is cough, which affects ~10% of subjects. The cough is typically irritating, dry and non-productive and is not dose related. A number of suggestions have been put forward as to the aetiology of the cough including potentiation of bradykinin levels by ACE inhibition, an increased sensitivity of the normal cough reflex, and finally increased levels of circulating prostaglandins. However, the cough is definitely due to inhibition of ACE rather than the blockade of the renin–angiotensin system, as angiotensin II receptor antagonists do not exhibit this side-effect.

As previously mentioned, first-dose hypotension is a side-effect of ACE inhibition which is especially common in subjects on high doses of diuretics. Acute renal failure can also result when patients with unrecognized renal artery stenosis are given ACE inhibitor therapy and also in subjects with pre-existing renal disease taking non-steroidal anti-inflammatory drugs.

Angio-oedema is a rare but potentially life-threatening side-effect of ACE inhibition. It commonly occurs within several days to a week after initiation of therapy. Interestingly it appears to be more common after treatment with combined ACE/neutral endopeptidase inhibition although the mechanism for this is unclear.

A macular rash is occasionally seen in 3–5% of cases. Finally, loss of taste and appetite is also an uncommon side-effect but it can occur especially in the elderly, leading to weight loss if the condition is not recognized. It may take up to 2 weeks for the symptoms to resolve completely.

7.33   What is the evidence-base for this class of drugs?

The evidence-base for ACE inhibitors is not extensive. There are no large randomized studies comparing ACE inhibition to placebo in patients with hypertension. However, a recent study (CAPP study) compared a regime based on the ACE inhibitor captopril with standard therapy based on diuretics and β-blockade. Although the study design has been questioned, outcomes were broadly similar between the groups, but there were significantly more strokes in the group treated with ACE inhibition (Hansson et al 1999b). Another recent study (STOP 2) also showed no clear benefit in terms of outcome of ACE inhibition over conventional therapy

(Hansson *et al* 1999a). In the CAPP study, subjects with coexisting type 2 diabetes appeared to obtain greater benefit in terms of reduction in cardiovascular disease endpoints than patients with diabetes on conventional therapy. However, this finding was not supported by results from the UKPDS comparing antihypertensive therapy with captopril or atenolol in a large cohort of newly diagnosed type 2 diabetics (UKPDS Group 1998). The most recent study to use ACE inhibitors was a large randomized placebo-controlled study that showed that addition of ramipril reduced cardiovascular events by 22% and death by 16% in a high-risk population, 50% of whom had hypertension (Yusuf *et al* 2000). However, it remains controversial as to whether the majority of the observed benefit was due to reduction in blood pressure or a blood pressure-independent effect of ACE inhibition.

7.34 What factors influence their efficacy?

The major factors influencing the efficacy of ACE inhibitors include ethnicity and the degree of activation of the renin–angiotensin system. Black African subjects with essential hypertension are more likely to exhibit volume-expanded, low-renin hypertension, and it has been shown that such subjects respond less well to therapy with ACE inhibition than matched white Caucasian subjects. Response of black African subjects can be improved by activation of the renin–angiotensin system by additional therapy with a diuretic. Indeed the response of white Caucasian subjects can also be improved by addition of a diuretic to their antihypertensive regime. It has also been suggested that an individual's ACE genotype may influence response to therapy, although the evidence for this hypothesis is not strong, and no large-scale trials have demonstrated such an effect of genotypes.

7.35 Is there a dose–response relationship?

Although there is some evidence to support a dose–response relationship, it is unclear whether a patient with an inadequate blood pressure response to ACE inhibition would benefit more from addition of a diuretic or an increased dose of ACE inhibition. Nevertheless, 'standard doses' such as 20 mg of lisinopril are usually employed (lower starting doses may be needed); higher doses may be used if there is a good response to ACE inhibition.

7.36 Are there differences between drugs in this class?

Most ACE inhibitors have similar actions, although they differ chemically, the major difference being the chemical group that interacts to block the active site of ACE. The first clinically available ACE inhibitor captopril has a sulphydryl group, which has been implicated in its side-effects such as taste disturbance, although this is not proven. Other ACE inhibitors such as enalapril and lisinopril have a carboxyl group, and the ACE inhibitor fosinopril has a fosphitinic acid group. The majority of ACE inhibitors are prodrugs (enalapril, quinopril, perindopril) being activated to their active form by metabolism in the liver. Some ACE inhibitors (captopril, lisinopril), however, are immediately active on absorption.

Finally, ACE inhibitors differ in duration of action and mode of excretion and thus in their frequency of administration. In terms of prevention of cardiovascular events, there is no evidence that any ACE inhibitor is superior to another and benefits are thus a class effect.

ANGIOTENSIN II RECEPTOR ANTAGONISTS

7.37 What are their mechanisms of action?

Unlike ACE inhibitors, angiotensin II receptor antagonists inhibit the renin–angiotensin system by blocking the action of angiotensin II at the level of the AT_1 receptor (*Fig. 7.5*). This receptor mediates virtually all the known biological actions of angiotensin II, so their effect is similar to ACE inhibition. However, there are a number of differences. ACE inhibition may fail to completely inhibit the renin–angiotensin system owing to the fact that angiotensin II may be produced via non-ACE-mediated pathways such as the chymase pathway. In addition, angiotensin II may be produced at a local level by pathways inaccessible to ACE inhibition. Finally, it has also been shown in some patients on long-term therapy with ACE inhibition that they exhibit the phenomenon of 'escape' and that angiotensin II can be measured in their circulation. Unlike ACE inhibitors, angiotensin II receptor antagonists do not potentiate circulating levels of bradykinin, which may be of benefit or not depending on whether the overall effect of bradykinin is beneficial or detrimental.

7.38 What are the indications for their use?

The major compelling indication for the use of an angiotensin II receptor antagonist is in subjects who experience a troublesome cough on ACE inhibitor therapy. Studies have convincingly shown that in patients with ACE inhibitor-induced cough, angiotensin II receptor antagonists do not cause cough. Other possible indications for their use would be coexisting heart failure or intolerance of other major classes of antihypertensive drug. The evidence-base for angiotensin II receptor antagonists being renoprotective is less strong than that for ACE inhibition. However, two recent studies demonstrated that angiotensin II receptor antagonism was able to protect against progression of nephropathy in subjects with type 2 diabetes (Lewis *et al* 2001) and that its effect on the development of diabetic nephropathy in patients with type 2 diabetes was independent of its blood pressure-lowering effect (Parving *et al* 2001).

7.39 What are the contraindications to their use?

 The contraindications for the use of angiotensin II receptor antagonists currently should be considered to be the same as those for ACE inhibition as outlined above (Q. 7.31).

7.40 What are their adverse effects?

 With the exception of cough, the adverse effects of angiotensin II receptor antagonists are similar to those of ACE inhibition. Nevertheless, angiooedema seems to be a rare side-effect.

α-BLOCKERS

7.41 What are the mechanisms of action?

The α-blockers act by inhibiting the postsynaptic α_1-adrenoceptors on vascular smooth muscle. This inhibits the vasoconstrictor effect of circulating and locally released catecholamines (adrenaline (epinephrine) and noradrenaline (norepinephrine)), resulting in peripheral vasodilatation.

7.42 What are the indications for their use?

Compelling indications for the use of α-blocking agents would be in men with symptoms of prostatism. A number of controlled trials have demonstrated increased urinary flow rates in hypertensive men with coexisting benign prostatic hyperplasia who are treated with α-blockers. There is also evidence from meta-analysis that treatment with α-blockers will decrease levels of total cholesterol, triglycerides and increase HDL levels slightly compared to other antihypertensive agents (Kasiske et al 1995). However, this is unlikely to have any major clinical benefit.

7.43 What are the contraindications for their use?

 A major contraindication to the use of α-blockade is urinary incontinence. α-blockers may worsen stress incontinence, especially in overweight women. α-blockers should also be used with care in individuals with postural hypotension, as they are likely to exacerbate it. If they are to be used, they should be given in low doses initially with instructions to take the first dose in bed in the evening.

7.44 What are their adverse effects?

 The major adverse effects of α-blockers are postural hypertension, tachycardia, dizziness, stress incontinence and gastrointestinal upset.

7.45   What is the evidence-base for these drugs?

The evidence-base for α-blockers is very small compared to that of agents such as diuretics and β-blockers. Until recently there were no trials based on α-blockade, which showed reduction in cardiovascular endpoints. Indeed the α-blocker doxazosin was recently withdrawn from the ALLHAT study because of a suggestion that there was increased incidence of heart failure in patients who were taking doxazosin (Messerli 2000). However, α-blockade with doxazosin is currently being assessed in a large hypertension study – the ASCOT study.

7.46   What factors influence their efficacy?

There is no evidence, to date, that α-blockers are more or less effective in any patient group, or between younger or older hypertensives. However, α-blockade is especially effective in the rare circumstance of a patient with catecholamine excess resulting from a phaeochromocytoma.

ARTERIAL VASODILATORS

7.47   What are their mechanisms of action?

Direct-acting vasodilators include hydralazine, minoxidil and diazoxide. Although hydralazine was used for many years as a third-line agent in combination with diuretics and β-blockers, its exact mechanism of action still remains unclear. It produces direct vasodilatation and is predominantly an arteriolar dilator rather than a venodilator. Tissue levels of hydralazine have been shown to correlate more accurately with its antihypertensive activity than circulating ones. Minoxidil and diazoxide are extremely potent vasodilators and work by activating potassium channels in vascular smooth muscle, leading to depolarization and relaxation.

7.48   What are the indications for their use?

Hydralazine is now very rarely used in the clinical management of essential hypertension. However, it is still occasionally used in treating hypertension associated with pregnancy, as there is no evidence that it is harmful to either the fetus or the mother.

Minoxidil is only indicated for patients who have proved refractory to treatment with all other hypertensive agents and is, therefore, now only rarely used in clinical practice.

Diazoxide, possibly the most potent vasodilator drug in use today, was originally used to lower blood pressure in hypertensive patients on renal dialysis (who had to be given very large fluid challenges). Diazoxide is now a drug used only rarely for patients with severe hypertension resistant to other agents.

7.49 What are the contraindications to their use?

Since direct vasodilators promote a reflex tachycardia, monotherapy with such agents would be contraindicated in patients with angina that was particularly rate dependent. However, in normal clinical practice it is nearly always necessary to co-administer a β-blocker with direct-acting vasodilator. Direct-acting vasodilators are also contraindicated as first-line agents, owing to their side-effect profile.

7.50 What are their adverse effects?

As a direct result of the extensive vasodilatation and decreased peripheral resistance and blood pressure that occur with direct-acting vasodilators, a number of physiological counter-regulatory mechanisms are activated. These include baroreceptor stimulation, tachycardia and release of catecholamines. Such effects lead to sodium retention and expansion of fluid volume, which limits the usefulness of direct-acting vasodilators as antihypertensives. A further limitation is due to the development of tachyphylaxis. In addition, the major side-effects that preclude their use as first-line agents, in addition to tachycardia and fluid retention, include flushing and headaches.

In the case of minoxidil, excessive hair growth on the face and body is especially troublesome in women. Because of the tachycardia and severe fluid retention, patients on minoxidil frequently need treatment with β-blockade and large doses of a potent diuretic; doses of furosemide (frusemide) as high as 200 mg a day may be necessary to prevent the massive fluid accumulation that may occur.

Treatment with hydralazine especially at high doses (100–150 mg b.d.) may cause a lupus-like syndrome. This is not usually very common but positive antinuclear antibodies may occur in up to 40% of patients on treatment. Symptoms include fever, rash and/or arthralgia and should resolve on stopping the drug. It has been suggested that subjects have a genetic predisposition to developing this syndrome when treated with hydralazine.

Diazoxide is diabetogenic owing to its chemical similarity to thiazide diuretics. Patients on chronic high doses may require therapy with oral hypoglycaemic agents.

7.51 What is the evidence-base for these drugs?

There is virtually no evidence-base for these drugs, as they have never been assessed in properly controlled randomized clinical trials. As discussed, they are often reserved for difficult-to-control patients who have failed to respond to therapy with other major classes of antihypertensive.

7.52 What factors influence their efficacy?

Direct-acting vasodilators are likely to be most efficacious in subjects in whom hypertension is particularly due to a large increase in peripheral vascular resistance.

7.53 Is there a dose–response relationship?

There is a dose–response relationship, but this also holds true for the side-effects associated with these agents. Moreover, in the case of hydralazine, it has been shown that the antihypertensive response correlates better with tissue rather than circulating hydralazine levels.

7.54 Are there differences between drugs in this class?

 The major side-effects and limitations to usage are similar among these drugs. Minoxidil and diazoxide both act by opening potassium channels and hydralazine is a direct-acting vasodilator. Whereas minoxidil causes excessive hair growth, diazoxide does not.

CENTRALLY ACTING DRUGS

7.55 What are their mechanisms of action?

Centrally acting drugs have their action in the vasomotor centres of the brain. They act primarily by stimulating α_2-receptors, leading to stimulation of inhibitory neurons and a decreased central sympathetic outflow. These effects cause a decrease in peripheral resistance and a decrease in cardiac output, which lowers blood pressure. Centrally acting drugs include α-methyldopa, clonidine, guanethidine and moxonidine (which is an imidazaline receptor agonist).

7.56 What are the indications for their use?

The clinical usage of these agents has decreased significantly, although a number of patients who have been on long-term antihypertensive therapy may still be taking them. Although there are no compelling evidence-based indications for the use of centrally acting agents, possible indications include type 1 diabetes, patients who have experienced side-effects with other major antihypertensive classes, and as a third-line agent in patients who have responded inadequately to other agents. Methyldopa is still used extensively in the treatment of hypertension in pregnancy and pre-eclampsia.

7.57 What are the contraindications to their use?

 The major contraindications to the use of these agents would be a previous history of depression or patients who drive or operate machinery, as drowsiness is a common side-effect.

7.58   What are their adverse effects?

 Side-effects occur commonly with these agents and dropout rates can be as high as 30%. The major common side-effects include sedation, dry mouth, drowsiness, dizziness, fatigue, headaches, depression and vivid dreams. Symptoms of depression are often subtle, especially in the elderly, and include decreased mental agility and a lack of the ability to enjoy life. Moreover, studies have shown that quality of life assessments decrease further when a diuretic is added to a centrally acting agent.

7.59   What is the evidence base for this class of drugs?

As with direct-acting vasodilators, there is no established evidence-base for these agents, especially with regard to cardiovascular outcome.

OTHER ANTIHYPERTENSIVE DRUGS

7.60   Can nitrates be used to lower blood pressure?

Nitrates cause vasodilatation by releasing nitric oxide (NO). Recently NO produced locally by the blood vessel wall has been shown, at least in part, to regulate arterial stiffness. Since older subjects with isolated systolic hypertension (ISH) frequently have increased stiffness of the large arteries as a cause of their blood pressure rather than an increase in peripheral resistance, nitrates are likely to be of particular benefit in patients with ISH. Indeed, a recent trial, using the long-acting nitrate isosorbide mononitrate convincingly demonstrated significant reduction of blood pressure in a cohort of subjects with ISH (Stokes & Ryan 1997).

7.61   Do antioxidants lower blood pressure?

Recent data from the Third National Health and Nutritional Examination Survey (NHANES III) demonstrated a clear correlation between lower blood pressure and increasing levels of antioxidants such as beta-carotene and vitamin C in 15 142 US subjects. Interestingly, the same study suggested that vitamin E levels may be associated with higher blood pressure. However, the majority of epidemiological studies also support a relationship between increased antioxidant levels and lower blood pressure. However, as yet, no large double-blind, randomized, placebo-controlled studies have been undertaken. Nevertheless, several, but not all, small human studies have shown reduction in blood pressure in subjects with essential hypertension treated with antioxidant vitamins (Kitiyakara & Wilcox 1998). Further studies have also suggested that addition of antioxidants to drug-based antihypertensive regimes may also be effective in further blood pressure reduction, although this has not been confirmed in large studies.

The mechanisms whereby antioxidants reduce blood pressure remain unclear, although a number of suggestions have been put forward, including blockade of the action of angiotensin II, inhibition of serum ACE activity and improvement in vascular endothelial function. Recent evidence would suggest that properly randomized trials should be undertaken to address the effect of various antioxidant vitamins on blood pressure.

7.62   Does fish oil lower blood pressure?

Original interest focused on the effects of dietary n-6 fatty acids derived from vegetable oils, which had been reported to lower blood pressure and, in addition, decrease platelet aggregation and reduce clinical events leading to vascular occlusion. Since polyunsaturated fatty acids influence the production of prostaglandins and eicosanoids, they can affect many physiological processes involved in the regulation of blood pressure. A controlled study of n-3 fatty acid supplementation given as fish oil, demonstrated a clear 6.5 mmHg reduction in systolic blood pressure and 4.4 mmHg reduction in diastolic blood pressure in subjects with essential hypertension (Knapp & FitzGerald 1989). Subsequent studies have also demonstrated that fish oil supplementation decreases blood pressure in essential hypertension (Howe 1997). The most likely mechanism of action is a decrease in constrictor prostanoids and an increase in dilator prostanoids. However, since fish oil also alters the fatty acid composition of cell membranes, it may also lower blood pressure by altering the activity of the membrane sodium transport systems. Fish oil has also been used in an attempt to reduce blood pressure in pregnancy-induced hypertension, but benefit has not been clearly demonstrated in this situation. Whether addition of fish oil to existing antihypertensive therapy would provide additional blood pressure reduction also remains to be tested.

7.63   Do statins reduce blood pressure?

Statins reduce the incidence of stroke by around 32% in a meta-analysis of the lipid-lowering trials, despite the fact that there is as yet no epidemiological evidence of a link between cholesterol and thrombotic stroke. However, there is clear evidence of a link between blood pressure and stroke, and blood pressure reduction results in a similar (40%) reduction in stroke. These findings have led investigators to suggest that treatment with statins may decrease blood pressure and this may mediate to a large extent their reduction in stroke. Recently the hypotensive effect of statin therapy was clearly demonstrated in a trial involving the use of pravastatin in subjects with hypercholesterolaemia and essential hypertension (Glorioso et al 2000). Interestingly, fibrate therapy in subjects with hypertriglyceridaemia has also been recently shown to be associated with a reduction in blood pressure. Since many hypertensives have coexisting hypercholesterolaemia, it may be that statin therapy may have the additional benefit of blood pressure lowering in addition to its hypocholesterolaemic effect. However, it will be important to test this hypothesis in large properly controlled randomized studies.

 PATIENT QUESTIONS

7.64 Can hypertension be cured?

In the vast majority of cases high blood pressure cannot be cured, and life-long therapy is required. The aim of the therapy is to reduce the blood pressure and thus the risks associated with hypertension (*see Ch. 1*). Stopping therapy invariably leads to a rise in blood pressure and cannot be recommended for most patients.

7.65 Do I have to take drugs?

Most people will require drug therapy to control their elevated blood pressure. However, in the majority of patients it is often wise to try non-drug measures first, before drugs are initiated. Weight loss in obese people can lead to a fall in blood pressure, as can a reduction in alcohol and salt intake in most subjects. However, it is wise to discuss such measures with your GP first before embarking on radical lifestyle changes. One should also realize that such measures are likely only to lead to a modest reduction in blood pressure (10 mmHg at most). Finally, stopping smoking is the most important thing to attempt, as it has the most impact on risk.

 ### 7.66 Don't drugs have side-effects?

No drug is without side-effects. However, the vast majority of modern drugs are well tolerated and only cause problems in a small minority of patients. Sometimes side-effects can be intolerable and require the medication to be withdrawn. However, as with any treatment, it is important to weigh up the benefits of treatment against the risks and inconvenience. All medications now come with a patient information leaflet which lists all the likely side-effects, although some of them will be vanishingly rare.

7.67 Do herbal remedies reduce blood pressure?

There is no hard evidence from placebo-controlled trials that herbal medicines reduce blood pressure, and certainly no evidence that they decrease the risk of strokes or heart attacks. Nevertheless, antioxidants and fish oil supplements can reduce blood pressure slightly and may help in people with borderline high blood pressure. However, they are no substitute for a healthy diet rich in fish, fruit and vegetables.

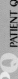

Targets, multiple risk intervention and compliance

TREATMENT TARGETS

8.1 What are appropriate blood pressure targets?

The recommended target blood pressures, based on the current British Hypertension Society Guidelines, for treated hypertensive patients are summarized in Table 8.1. These recognize the increased risk among diabetic patients, and acknowledge trial evidence that adhering to particularly tight blood pressure control in this group is associated with improved outcome.

8.2 What is the evidence for the targets?

Evidence for these recommended targets is largely obtained from the Hypertension Optimal Treatment (HOT) study (Hansson *et al* 1998), which was designed to study the effects on outcome of lowering blood pressure to three distinct diastolic targets, ≤90 mmHg, ≤85 mmHg and ≤80 mmHg (*Fig. 8.1*). It should be noted that systolic blood pressure ≤140 mmHg was achieved in all patients assigned to the latter group. The HOT study clearly demonstrated that the risk of myocardial infarction and cardiovascular mortality could be minimized by attaining the currently recommended blood pressure targets. Furthermore, in diabetic hypertensive patients there appeared to be a significant advantage in reducing blood pressure below the optimal blood pressure for non-diabetics.

TABLE 8.1 Treated blood pressure targets recommended by the British Hypertension Society, where 'audit standard' reflects the minimum recommended level of blood pressure control

	Clinic BP (mmHg)		Mean daytime ABPM or home BP	
	No diabetes	Diabetes	No diabetes	Diabetes
Optimal BP	<140/85	<140/80	<130/80	<130/75
Audit standard	<150/90	<140/85	<140/85	<140/80

From Ramsay *et al* 1999, with permission of the Nature Publishing Group.

8.3 Is there a 'J'-shaped curve?

There is ongoing debate over the apparent association with increased mortality of lower extremes of blood pressure. Several factors underlie the appearance of such J-shaped curves during antihypertensive treatment. Firstly, very small numbers actually achieve very low treated systolic and diastolic blood pressures, which is evidenced by the wide standard error

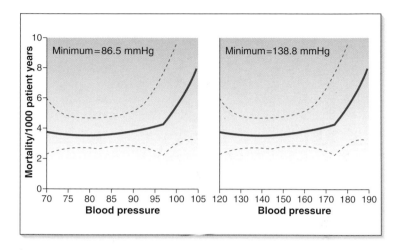

Fig. 8.1 Effect of different levels of blood pressure control in the HOT study. Cardiovascular mortality per 1000 patient-years in the hypertension optimal treatment (HOT) study, which demonstrated optimal treated blood pressure targets. (From Hansson *et al* 1998, with permission of Elsevier Science.)

margins around this part of the curve, as seen in Figure 8.1, and this makes statistical interpretation difficult. Among those patients with significantly lower than optimal blood pressure will be a significant proportion in whom hypotension is a consequence of concurrent illness, for example congestive cardiac failure, rather than antihypertensive treatment. The association with increased risk appears strongest for very low diastolic rather than systolic pressure, and this is consistent with our understanding that large artery stiffness, which is characterized by high systolic blood pressure and low diastolic blood pressure, is itself associated with heightened cardiovascular risk. In particular, very low diastolic pressures may impair coronary artery perfusion and thus precipitate or worsen myocardial ischaemia. However, there is no direct evidence that, in patients with cerebrovascular or cardiovascular disease, maximal blood pressure reduction could precipitate rather than prevent atherosclerotic disease complications.

8.4 Can targets be achieved?

In light of new evidence of potential advantages, we are striving to achieve lower blood pressure targets than in the past. Despite this, data from several studies, including the HOT study have shown that stepwise antihypertensive titration allows blood pressure targets to be achieved in the majority of patients (*Fig. 8.2*). Although this study focused on diastolic

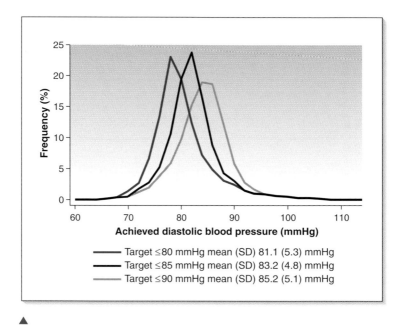

Fig. 8.2 Distribution of mean diastolic blood pressures achieved in the Hypertension Optimal Treatment (HOT) study. Note that the majority of patients achieved target blood pressure in each group. From Hansson *et al* 1998, with permission.

blood pressure targets, and more than 90% of patients achieved a diastolic blood pressure of ≤90 mmHg, all of the group assigned to tightest blood pressure control achieved systolic blood pressure of ≤160 mmHg.

8.5 Does blood pressure reduction normalize risk?

Whilst there is good evidence that blood pressure reduction reduces risk, it is unclear to what extent risk can be completely normalized. Several recent population-based studies have reported survival among treated hypertensive patients compared to non-hypertensive controls. One such study from Malmo in Sweden demonstrated that the risk of myocardial infarction in elderly hypertensive men, who had attained target diastolic blood pressures ≤90 mmHg, was four times higher than in their non-hypertensive counterparts (*Fig. 8.3*). Similar findings were identified in a Gothenburg population study where, in addition, systolic blood pressure was controlled to ≤160 mmHg. There exists a wide margin of risk between treated hypertensive patients and non-hypertensive individuals and, therefore, risk does not appear to be normalized. It could be suggested, however, that

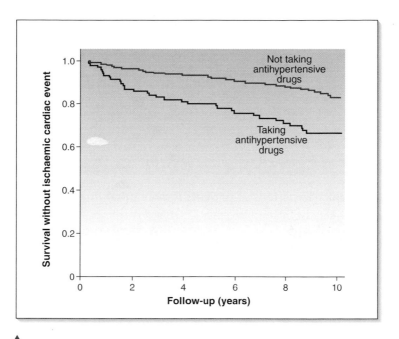

▲

Fig. 8.3 Risk amongst treated hypertensives. Survival curves among treated hypertensive patients and non-hypertensive individuals from the Malmo population study. (From Merlo *et al* 1996, with permission of the BMJ Publishing Group.)

treatment in these studies was less likely to normalize risk, owing to less stringent blood pressure targets. Moreover, these studies suggest that in hypertensive patients blood pressure control alone is insufficient to achieve maximal risk reduction, and emphasize the importance of other measures to reduce global cardiovascular risk (*see* Qs 8.7–8.10).

8.6   Can therapy be withdrawn?

Antihypertensive drug withdrawal has been considered in observational studies and randomized controlled trials for patients with established and controlled blood pressure. In the majority of cases, blood pressure rises to pretreatment levels or higher, and, in a smaller number of cases, blood pressure rises to a lesser value than pretreatment pressure (Fletcher *et al* 1988). In a small number of patients, blood pressure appears to remain controlled despite withdrawal of antihypertensive medication. However, few of these patients remain normotensive if followed up, for example <15% at 1 year. Indeed, it is likely that most of the normotensive individuals have been incorrectly diagnosed because of several atypical blood pressure readings, or that body habits or other lifestyle factors have been positively modified in the interim. There is no apparent disease-modifying effect of antihypertensive therapy, insofar as it appears to exert effects on blood pressure only for the duration of its administration.

MULTIPLE RISK FACTOR INTERVENTION

8.7 Which hypertensive patients require other interventions?

As discussed above, blood pressure reduction reduces, but fails to normalize, cardiovascular risk. Therefore, certain hypertensive patients may benefit from other interventions to reduce overall risk, and those at highest overall risk are identified by the presence of established cardiovascular disease, or have ≥15% 10-year coronary heart disease risk as determined by cardiac risk assessment (*see Ch. 5*).

8.8 Is cholesterol reduction important?

In order to achieve maximal widespread cardiovascular risk reduction, cholesterol-lowering treatment is targeted to those at highest cardiovascular risk (*Box 8.1*). These current recommendations take account of several issues, including pharmacoeconomic implications of treatment, and are likely to be conservative and, therefore, should be regarded as the minimum acceptable threshold for treatment. This is emphasized by the recent

---

BOX 8.1 Factors prompting statin treatment in hypertensive patients

■ Serum total cholesterol ≥5.0 mmol/l*

AND

■ *Familial hypercholesterolaemia*
■ *Secondary prevention:* myocardial infarction, CABG or angioplasty, cerebrovascular disease, peripheral vascular disease, atherosclerotic renovascular disease
■ *Primary prevention:* 10-year CHD risk ≥15% as per the Cardiac Risk Assessor

---

* This may have to be revised in light of the data from the Heart Protection Study, which will be available shortly.

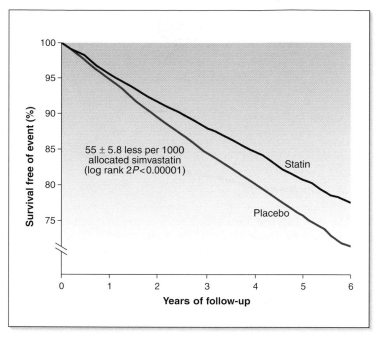

▲

Fig. 8.4 Effect of cholesterol reduction. The Heart Protection Study showed that in patients with hypertension, coronary artery disease, peripheral vascular disease or diabetes, and cholesterol >3.5 mmol/l statin treatment led to 55 fewer vascular events per 1000 patients treated. (Provisional results published with kind permission of the Heart Protection Study Cohaborative Group, http://www.hpsinfo.org)

findings of the Heart Protection Study, which studied the effects of statin treatment in patients with hypertension, coronary heart disease, peripheral arterial disease or diabetes mellitus who had total cholesterol >3.5 mmol/l. Treatment was associated with a substantial reduction in vascular events (*Fig. 8.4*).

8.9 Which hypertensives should receive aspirin?

There is some contention over the value of aspirin treatment in hypertensive patients. The Thrombosis Prevention Trial was a placebo-controlled study of the effects of 75 mg daily aspirin, or warfarin, and 26% of the study population were hypertensive. Aspirin led to a 16% reduction in all cardiovascular events, 20% reduction in myocardial infarction, and no effect on fatal events (*Fig. 8.5*). The number of events prevented was offset by similar rates for adverse bleeding events. These findings were similar to

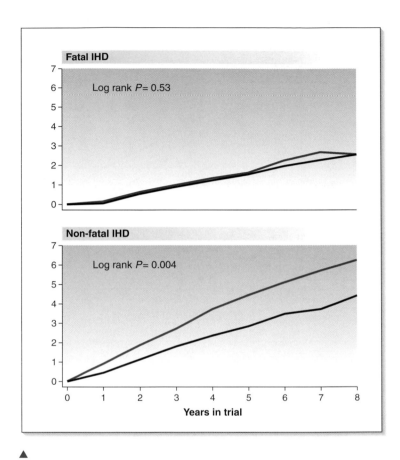

Fig. 8.5 Effect of aspirin. Cumulative proportion (%) of men with ischaemic heart disease (IHD) in the Thrombosis Prevention Trial (open circles on aspirin, closed circles on placebo). (From Medical Research Council's General Practice Research Framework 1998, with permission of Elsevier Science.)

an arm of the Hypertension Optimal Treatment (HOT) study, which compared 75 mg daily aspirin to placebo. Most bleeding events occurred in patients with particularly high systolic blood pressures. Based on these studies, the optimal use of aspirin in hypertensive patients is summarized in Box 8.2.

> ### BOX 8.2 Guidance for the use of aspirin in hypertension
>
> No contraindication to aspirin
> - *Secondary prevention:* established cerebrovascular disease, coronary artery disease, peripheral vascular disease or atherosclerotic renovascular disease
>
> OR
>
> - *Primary prevention* (blood pressure must be controlled to <150/90 AND age ≥ 50 years):
>   - target organ damage (e.g. LVH, renal impairment or proteinuria), OR
>   - 10-year CHD risk ≥ 15% by cardiac risk assessment, OR
>   - type 2 diabetes mellitus

8.10 Do normotensives at high risk benefit from blood pressure lowering?

The definition of hypertension is somewhat arbitrary, and it would appear that the risk reduction associated with blood pressure lowering is continuous. Therefore, benefits may be observed by lowering blood pressure, even when it may appear to be 'normal'. These benefits are particularly evident in patients with highest absolute cardiovascular risk; for example, the HOPE study (Yusuf *et al* 2000) demonstrated that even a modest reduction in blood pressure by an ACE inhibitor led to a very significant reduction in cardiovascular events in patients unselected for blood pressure with high risk, including those with established coronary artery disease, peripheral vascular disease, and diabetes mellitus. It is possible that some of the observed benefits were due to properties of ACE inhibitors other than blood pressure reduction, although this remains subject to some speculation.

COMPLIANCE WITH TREATMENT

8.11 How big a problem is poor compliance?

Non-compliance may account for up to half of all cases where there is apparent failure of medical therapy in hypertension (Stephenson 1999). Several reports have indicated that blood pressure is maintained at target levels in as few as 30% of patients, and it is likely that compliance is an important factor contributing to these poor figures. Compliance is often overlooked, and physicians tend to escalate the prescribed dose or add on further antihypertensive drugs unnecessarily. It is estimated that prescribing physician estimates of compliance are reasonable for patients with good compliance, but miss non-compliance in about two-thirds of cases.

8.12 What factors influence compliance?

Compliance can be defined as the adherence by the patient to directions given by the prescribing physician, where good compliance is generally considered at the 80% level or greater. Attitudes are the best predictor of regular compliance, while drug-related symptoms appear to be the best predictor of non-compliance. It is mainly subjective criteria that influence compliance, for example perception of hypertension and its treatment, the doctor and environment. Important factors include patient follow-up with reiteration of administration directions, and use of simplified dosing regimens, for example once-daily preparations and medications taken in the morning (Mallion *et al* 1998). To minimize the tendency for non-compliance as far as possible, drugs with favourable side-effect profiles and regimens with minimal adverse drug interaction are preferred.

8.13 How can compliance be assessed?

Direct patient questioning is notoriously unreliable; however, quality of life questionnaires may be important in determining the effects of a particular antihypertensive drug, or regimen, on subjective sense of well-being. Tablet counts provide slightly better objective evidence, although these can also be misleading and give no indication of dosing pattern. Blood drug concentrations can be measured and, in certain cases, this can be used to confirm non-compliance; however, these tests are often difficult to obtain and are unable to establish whether patients adhere correctly to any given regimen. More recently, electronic devices that record the time when tablet containers are opened have offered the opportunity for better objective patients assessment (Mallion *et al* 1998) (*Fig. 8.6*). They have been used to show that, even in the setting of a clinical trial, 30–40% of patients substantially underdose because of non-compliance, compared with 7–10% as pill-counts falsely indicate. In exceptional cases, where there is a strong degree of suspicion, a period of inpatient drug administration with observation of blood pressure may be required.

8.14 How can compliance be improved?

Certain interventions have been shown to be successful in improving compliance, particularly re-enforcement and encouragement. For example, in a patient group who were taught how to measure their own blood-pressure and pill taking, and taught how to tailor pill taking to their usual daily routine there was a reported improvement in compliance of 21.3% (1.5% in a non-intervention placebo group), associated with a fall in blood pressure in 85% of patients (56% in placebo group) (Haynes *et al* 1976). Simple dosing regimens are important, and those that involve more than twice-daily dosing are reported to have a consistently higher rate of non-

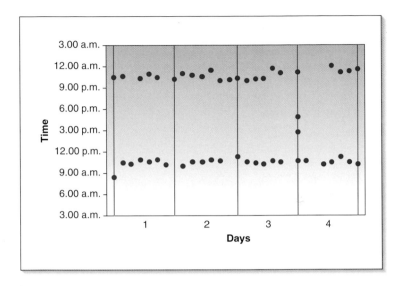

Fig. 8.6 An example of how electronic monitoring can be used to assess patients' tablet-taking behaviour. A microchip records each time the container is opened and closed. In this case, there is good compliance (>80% adherence) with a twice-daily preparation. (From Stephenson *et al* 1999, with permission of the American Medical Association.)

compliance. Polypharmacy should be avoided for similar reasons, underlining the importance of adhering to effective and rational drug combinations associated with as few major adverse effects as possible. It is important to counsel patients on the possible short-term adverse symptoms that may be due to the effects of blood pressure lowering per se, which is often most important in the first few weeks after treatment initiation. This may avoid the inappropriate early self-discontinuation of an otherwise effective antihypertensive therapy by the patient. Other measures to improve compliance include better psychological guidance for the patient, considering the individual patient's personality.

8.15 Do once-a-day regimens improve compliance?

There is clearer evidence that regimens that require dosing three or even four times daily are associated with poorer compliance. However, there is some contention over whether there is a significant compliance advantage offered by once-daily compared to twice-daily preparations. This has not yet been demonstrated unequivocally, and furthermore, there are concerns that some 24-hour-duration products may be less forgiving of doses that are missed or delayed by several hours. For some patients in whom there is significant polypharmacy, once-daily preparations may offer a simpler dosing regimen and encourage compliance for this reason, for example where several medicines might be taken together in the morning. However, there is currently no strong evidence that once-daily regimens offer any distinct advantage for most patients, and given that many are more costly preparations, they cannot be advocated more broadly.

Secondary hypertension

9

INTRODUCTION

9.1 How often is a cause for hypertension identified?

The vast majority of patients presenting with hypertension will be classified as having essential (primary) hypertension. Nevertheless, one should always consider the possibility of an underlying cause – *secondary hypertension*. Estimates of the frequency of secondary hypertension vary, owing to differences in case mix, screening investigations used, and local referral practice. However, an underlying cause can be identified in ~5–10% of hypertensives.

9.2 What are the causes of secondary hypertension?

The main causes of secondary hypertension are listed in Box 9.1.

BOX 9.1 Causes of secondary hypertension

Renal (~50%)
- Renal parenchymal disease (two-thirds)
  - Acute glomerular nephritis
  - Chronic glomerular nephritis
  - Others, e.g. polycystic kidney disease
- Renovascular (one-third)
  - Atheroma
  - Fibromuscular dysplasia
  - Others, e.g. thromboembolism, aortic dissection

Endocrine (20%)
- Hyperaldosteronism
  - Conn's syndrome (two-thirds)
  - Bilateral adrenal hyperplasia (one-third)
  - Carcinoma (rare)
- Cushing's syndrome
- Congenital adrenal hyperplasia
- Phaeochromocytoma
- Acromegaly
- Hyperparathyroidism
- Hyper- or hypothyroidism

Other
- Coarctation
- Pregnancy
  - Pre-eclampsia
  - Pregnancy-associated hypertension   *Continued over*

- Drugs
  - Oral contraceptive pill
  - Steroids
  - Ciclosporin
  - Erythropoietin
  - Cocaine, sympathomimetics, and others
- Polycythaemia rubra vera
- Paget's disease

Monogenic forms (rare) (see Qs 9.57–61)
- Syndrome of apparent mineralocorticoid excess
- Glucocorticoid-remediable aldosteronism
- Liddle's syndrome
- Gordon's syndrome

9.3 Who is most likely to have secondary hypertension?

Secondary hypertension is relatively more common in younger individuals, and those with 'resistant' hypertension. Sometimes there may be 'clues' to an underlying disorder, such as hypokalaemia or active urinary sediment. However, secondary hypertension may present at any age. Therefore, it is important always to consider the possibility of an underlying cause, since identification offers the chance of a cure; with freedom from the daily task of tablet taking and a significant reduction in cardiovascular risk.

RENAL PARENCHYMAL DISEASE

9.4 What are the main causes of renal parenchymal disease?
See Box 9.2.

BOX 9.2 Renal parenchymal disorders
- Acute and chronic glomerular nephritis
- Interstitial nephritis
- Pyelonephritis
- Nephrocalcinosis
- Polycystic kidney disease
- Renal tumours
- Renin-producing tumours
- Diabetes
- Obstruction
- Trauma

9.5 Who is likely to have renal disease?

 A number of conditions predispose to renal disease. Individuals who have congenitally abnormal urinary tracts, or who have been subject to frequent urinary tract infections during childhood, are particularly at risk of renal disease. Subjects with diabetes, especially if associated with poorly controlled hypertension, are also more likely to develop renal disease, due to either diabetic or hypertensive nephropathy, or often a combination of both. Polycystic kidneys are inherited as an autosomal dominant trait with incomplete penetrance. Therefore, if they are identified, relatives should be screened for the condition using abdominal ultrasound and, if it is present, should be followed up with regular blood pressure and renal function tests, as they are especially likely to develop hypertension and renal impairment.

The collagen vascular disorders such as polyarteritis nodosa, systemic lupus erythematosus (SLE) and Wegner's disease are also associated with renal disease as a manifestation of the systemic condition. Amyloidosis is also associated with renal disease as are renal calculi. Finally, the possibility of drug-induced renal disease (e.g. NSAIDs) should be considered.

9.6 What are the symptoms and signs of renal disease?

Early symptoms of renal disease may be non-specific and relate to uraemia, such as tiredness, nausea, vomiting and general malaise (*see Box 9.3*). There may also be specific features related to the underlying disease, e.g. rashes, nailfold infarcts, joint pains etc.

BOX 9.3 Signs and symptoms of renal disease

Signs
- Fluid retention
- Haematuria
- Hypertension
- Anaemia
- Hyperkalaemia
- Proteinuria

Symptoms
- Tiredness
- General malaise
- Nausea
- Vomiting
- Renal colic

9.7   What investigations should be undertaken?

Investigations in patients with renal disease are directed at ascertaining the severity of renal impairment and secondly at identifying the cause. The severity of renal disease can be assessed by measuring urinary 24-hour creatinine clearance. It should be noted that an accurate 24-hour urine collection is vital. Using the reciprocal plot of serum creatinine is also useful, as it will estimate when renal function will deteriorate to a stage where dialysis will be necessary. This allows for adequate discussion and preparation of the patient for this important step.

Routine biochemical tests including urea, creatinine, electrolytes, calcium and phosphate should be assessed. The full blood count should also be measured, as anaemia is common in patients with renal disease and can be corrected by treatment with erythropoietin. Inflammatory markers (CRP, ESR) and autoantibodies (e.g. ANA, ANCA) may also be helpful.

In patients with proteinuria but normal urea and creatinine, 24-hour urinary protein excretion should be measured and if this is excessive then a renal biopsy is sometimes necessary to diagnose conditions such as minimal change glomerulonephropathy. In addition, conditions associated with nephropathy such as diabetes and hypertension should be carefully assessed. A urine sample should be taken to look for cells, bacteria and active sediment. This should help to assess whether there is an element of acute inflammation with or without a specific cause.

9.8   What are the benefits of blood pressure reduction?

Blood pressure reduction is extremely beneficial in patients with renal parenchymal disease irrespective of its aetiology. There is a large evidence-base demonstrating that tight blood pressure control slows the decline of glomerular filtration rate (GFR) and decreases proteinuria in patients with renal disease.

9.9   Should ACE inhibitors be avoided?

ACE inhibitors are contraindicated in patients with renal artery stenosis (*see Qs 9.23*). However, once this condition has been excluded by appropriate investigation, ACE inhibitors are the drugs of choice in patients with diabetic nephropathy. This is because there is conclusive evidence that ACE inhibition is more effective at slowing the progression of diabetic renal disease than other antihypertensive agents that produce a similar reduction in blood pressure. Therefore ACE inhibitors appear to produce protective effects on renal function over and above simply lowering blood pressure although the mechanism is not fully clear. The evidence for ACE inhibitors being superior to other antihypertensives that produce similar decreases in blood pressure is far less clear in other forms of renal disease.

9.10   Are antihypertensive drugs less effective in renal disease?

PATIENTS WITH CREATININE CLEARANCE >25 ML/MIN

Antihypertensive therapy for patients within this group differs little from therapy in patients with normal renal function. The majority of these patients will respond to normal doses and combinations of antihypertensive agents. Therefore, any antihypertensive regimen should reflect the aetiology of the hypertension and any associated medical disorders.

PATIENTS WITH CREATININE CLEARANCE BETWEEN 5 AND 25 ML/MIN

Drug requirements are often increased at this level of renal impairment, and side-effects often limit the selection of antihypertensive agents. Thiazide diuretics are relatively ineffective at this degree of renal impairment (*see Q. 7.13*) and furosemide (frusemide) at doses of up to 50 mg/day or metolazone up to 30 mg/day should be used.

PATIENTS ON DIALYSIS

With the exception of diuretics, the antihypertensives used before the patient was placed on dialysis can be continued. Finally, a recent study in patients with end-stage renal failure showed that survival was improved in patients who had not only achieved blood pressure reduction, but had a reduction in large artery stiffness as measured by aortic pulse wave velocity. Therefore, antihypertensive agents of the future may be of greater benefit in renal disease, if in addition to lowering blood pressure they decrease arterial stiffness.

9.11   Which drugs should be used in the management of hypertension?

With the exception of thiazide diuretics, which have a reduced efficacy in patients with severe renal impairment, all the other classes of antihypertensive agents can be used in patients with renal disease. The choice of agent is normally determined by tolerability and coexisting medical conditions. In patients with creatinine clearance between 5 and 25 ml/min, side-effects often impose greater restrictions on the selection of agent used. As stated previously, diabetic nephropathy is a compelling indication to use an ACE inhibitor.

9.12   Is dose adjustment necessary?

Dose adjustment is often necessary and depends on a number of factors including the degree of renal impairment and the amount of drug excreted normally by the kidneys. This may necessitate a reduction in dose and a change in the dose interval. For patients with creatinine clearance >25 ml/min, dose adjustment is not often required.

9.13   What is the target blood pressure?

The British Hypertension Society guidelines recommend a threshold of systolic blood pressure ≥ 140 mmHg or a diastolic pressure of ≥ 90 mmHg for patients with persistent proteinuria or renal impairment. Optimal blood pressure control is $<130/85$ mmHg and reducing blood pressure to $<125/75$ mmHg may produce additional benefit in patients with chronic renal disease of any aetiology and proteinuria of ≥ 1 g/24 hours especially in diabetes.

9.14   Are patients with renal failure at high risk?

Patients with renal failure are at very high risk of cardiovascular disease and may need aspirin or statin therapy in addition to non-pharmacological measures to decrease their cardiovascular risk. Recently, increased arterial stiffness was shown to predict cardiovascular events and mortality in a large cohort of patients with end-stage renal failure. The patients, in whom both blood pressure and arterial stiffness were reduced, showed a decreased mortality compared to patients who despite blood pressure reduction had an increase in arterial stiffness. Future antihypertensive agents, which reduce arterial stiffness, may be of particular benefit in patients with renal failure.

9.15   Does haemodialysis reduce blood pressure?

Dialysis whether haemo- or peritoneal controls hypertension when present in 65–75% of cases. Of the remaining 25–35%, most can be controlled by aggressive use of antihypertensive agents.

9.16   Does transplantation cure hypertension?

Following renal transplantation, a patient's requirement for antihypertensive agents changes dramatically and a reduction in antihypertensive drugs may be required immediately following surgery, especially in patients who exhibit significant diuresis. Once stable renal function has been achieved, many patients may no longer need drug therapy. However, a significant number of transplant patients do still require antihypertensive therapy (Jacquot *et al* 1978), and this may be partly due to immunosuppressive regimens (*see Q. 9.17*). However, even in these patients, requirements for antihypertensive therapy may decrease over time and they should be identified and carefully followed up.

9.17   Does ciclosporin cause hypertension?

 There is good evidence that in some patients, ciclosporin does cause hypertension. The mechanisms involved are unclear but may be due to impairment of endothelial function or a direct effect on the renal vasculature.

9.18 How should ciclosporin-induced hypertension be managed?

The antihypertensive agent nifedipine has been shown to be effective in managing hypertension due to ciclosporin. Treatment with nifedipine has the additional advantage of allowing decreased doses of ciclosporin to be used on renal units, cutting costs significantly. This is because ciclosporin is metabolized via the cytochrome P450 system, which is inhibited by nifedipine. Thus co-administration of these drugs allows lower doses of ciclosporin to be used without loss of efficacy. Indeed, use of nifedipine is now common policy on most major renal units.

RENAL ARTERY STENOSIS

9.19 What are the causes of renal artery stenosis?

The commonest cause of renal artery stenosis is atherosclerotic renal disease, which accounts for approximately two-thirds of all cases (*Fig. 9.1*). The underlying pathology and risk factors for renal atherosclerosis are identical to those of atherosclerotic plaques elsewhere in the body. Indeed, atherosclerosis is invariably a systemic disorder, and it is unusual to find renal atheroma without accompanying lesions in the aorta. Most lesions occur in the main renal artery, but ostial lesions, which are difficult to treat, are often associated with advanced disease of the abdominal aorta. Bilateral disease occurs in ~ 25% of subjects.

Fibromuscular dysplasia accounts for most of the remaining cases of renal artery stenosis. It tends to affect the distal two-thirds of the renal artery and its branches, and can involve any layer of the arterial wall, but the medial form is most common. The aetiology is unknown. Other causes are listed in Box 9.4.

9.20 Who is at risk of renal artery stenosis?

The typical patient with atherosclerotic renal artery disease is an elderly male cigarette smoker, often with signs of atherosclerosis elsewhere.

BOX 9.4 Causes of renal artery stenosis

- Atherosclerosis (two-thirds)
- Fibromuscular dysplasia (one-third)
- Renal artery dissection
- Thromboembolism
- Trauma
- Neurofibromatosis
- Vasculitis

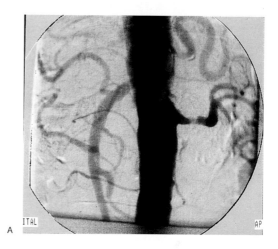

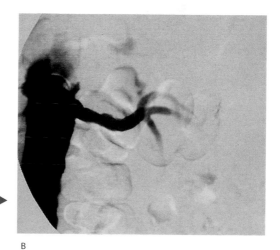

Fig. 9.1 Typical renal artery stenosis due to atheroma:
A. prior to angioplasty;
B. post-angioplasty.

Conversely, fibromuscular dysplasia tends to affect young females. However, not all renal artery lesions are clinically significant. Indeed, many patients with mild essential hypertension develop renal artery plaques without significantly compromising renal artery perfusion. Similarly, incidental moderate or severe renal artery lesions can be identified in normotensive individuals with normal renal function. Such issues cloud the figures relating to the incidence of renal artery stenosis and response to treatment, unless proof of the functional importance of a lesion is sought.

9.21 What are the symptoms and signs of renal artery stenosis?

Renal artery stenosis may be an asymptomatic disorder, and the only manifestation may be hypertension. However, subjects may present with 'resistant' or malignant hypertension, and even 'flash' pulmonary oedema (atherosclerotic disease). Clues to the diagnosis of renovascular disease include: renal impairment or deterioration in renal function after the introduction of an ACE inhibitor; loss of blood pressure control in a previously stable patient; and coexisting vascular disease. Other features may exist depending on the aetiology, e.g. rashes with renal artery vasculitis.

Physical signs are rarely helpful. By itself, an abdominal or renal bruit is of low predictive value, as they are common in the over-60s. However, a continuous abdominal bruit is a relatively good predictor of atherosclerotic renal disease, as is arterial disease in the legs.

Occlusion of the renal artery may be the presenting feature. Patients often complain of loin pain and haematuria, and may have hypertension and a fever.

9.22 How should patients be investigated for renal artery stenosis?

Besides assessing serum electrolytes and creatinine and blood pressure, a number of screening investigations for renal artery stenosis are currently available. Which one should be used depends to a large extent on availability and local experience (*see Box 9.5*). However, none is an ideal screening test and renal angiography remains the 'gold-standard'. Angiography allows lesions to be identified, localized and assessed for suitability of angioplasty or reconstructive surgery. Indeed, atherosclerotic lesions can be distinguished from fibromuscular dysplasia by angiography. Moreover, the pressure gradient across a lesion can be assessed, which may help in deciding whether treatment should be offered. However, angiography is not without its dangers. The contrast media used can lead to deterioration in renal function, and bleeding and dissection may occur as a complication of the instrumentation. Overall mortality is <0.1%, but complications can approach 3%, even in specialist centres. Therefore, a sensible approach may be to use screening tests when one has a moderate suspicion of renal artery disease, but opt directly for angiography when the index of suspicion is high (*Fig. 9.2*). MRI angiography may replace angiography as image resolution improves.

9.23 Are angiotensin-converting enzyme inhibitors contraindicated?

 In general angiotensin-converting enzyme inhibitors (ACEi) should be avoided in patients with significant renal artery stenosis, and should certainly not be used in patients with bilateral disease. Although they are

---

BOX 9.5 Screening tests for renal artery stenosis

Renal ultrasound

A disparity in kidney size can be a useful pointer to the presence of a renal artery lesion in the smaller kidney. Duplex scanning can also be used to assess blood flow. However, the technique is very operator-dependent and not suitable for all patients.

Captopril challenge

Plasma renin is measured before and 1 hour after 50 mg of captopril. Renin activity should rise if there is a significant lesion.

Renal vein renin

Simultaneous samples are taken from both renal veins and the inferior vena cava. A ratio >1.5 is taken as being positive. However, the test has relatively poor sensitivity and specificity, even if combined with salt loading or captopril.

Isotope renography

Alone, isotope renography is not sufficiently sensitive to identify significant renal artery lesions. However, when performed after administration of captopril, there is a significant improvement in sensitivity and specificity.

MRI angiography

This has limited availability, but image resolution is improving and it is non-invasive. It is, however, unable to provide information concerning the functional significance of lesions.

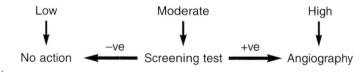

Fig. 9.2 Schema for investigation of suspected renal artery stenosis.

effective in reducing blood pressure, they may cause a marked and potentially irreversible reduction in renal function.

9.24 Is aspirin contraindicated?

Renal artery stenosis is not a contraindication to the use of aspirin. Indeed, in patients with atherosclerotic disease aspirin should be prescribed to reduce cardiovascular risk, unless there is a specific contraindication to its use.

9.25 Are non-steroidal anti-inflammatory drugs contraindicated?

Non-steroidal anti-inflammatory drugs should be used with caution in patients with renal artery stenosis as they may worsen both blood pressure control and renal function, especially if there is pre-existing renal impairment. If they are introduced then renal function should be monitored carefully.

9.26 Which drugs should be used?

Calcium-channel blockers are established as safe and effective for the treatment of hypertension in the majority of patients with renal artery disease. β-blockers may also be used, but may worsen the symptoms of peripheral vascular disease in some patients, especially if less β₁-selective agents are used. Angiotensin-converting enzyme inhibitors (ACEi) should be used with caution and avoided in bilateral disease (*see Q. 9.23*). Similarly, diuretics can exacerbate the hypovolaemia and hyponatraemia resulting from pressure natriuresis in the unaffected kidney. Moreover, thiazide diuretics are likely to be ineffective if there is significant renal impairment (*see Q. 7.10*).

9.27 Who should be offered renal angioplasty?

Predicting which patients are likely to benefit from angioplasty, with or without stenting, is difficult. Many centres only consider lesions >75% stenosis as likely to benefit. Although size is important in predicting the response to therapy, smaller lesions can be functionally significant, whereas larger ones may not be. Assessment of renal vein renin, the response of plasma renin to a captopril challenge, and the pressure gradient across a lesion may all help improve matters. Nevertheless, data from several studies suggest that angioplasty is more likely to be successful in controlling blood pressure and preventing a deterioration in renal function in young subjects who have not been hypertensive for long, and in subjects with fibromuscular dysplasia. It is least likely to be effective in older subjects with long-standing hypertension and widespread vascular disease. Indeed, one recent randomized trial suggested that there seems to be little advantage to renal artery angioplasty over medical therapy (van Jaarsveld *et al* 2000).

9.28 What is the success rate for angioplasty?

Technical success occurs in >70% of cases, and this is likely to improve with the widespread introduction of stenting. However, clinical success rates from angioplasty are much lower (Bonelli *et al* 1995). Approximately 50% of patients with fibromuscular dysplasia are cured (BP <140/90 off therapy), and in most of the remainder blood pressure control is substantially improved. Restenosis rates are low – around 5%. However, in older subjects with atherosclerotic disease, cure rates are typically <10%, with 50–60% of patients benefiting in terms of blood pressure control. Furthermore, angioplasty seems to have little effect on renal function, and carries a significant risk of complications, ~10–15% even in good centres, and restensosis rates are 20–30%, although these are likely to fall with the use of stents.

9.29 What are the risks of renal angioplasty?

Renal artery angioplasty is associated with a range of complications including: contrast nephropathy, renal artery dissection, embolization, haemorrhage, and haematoma formation. The risk of complications approaches ~10% even in good centres with a 30-day mortality of ~2.2% (Bonelli *et al* 1995).

9.30 Is surgery indicated?

Nephrectomy is now rarely performed for renal artery stenosis, and in general is only undertaken after angioplasty has failed. It should only be considered when the affected kidney is contributing <10% of total renal clearance, and is established as driving the hypertension. Success rates vary: ~20–50%. Surgical reconstruction of the diseased renal artery can also be undertaken. This may be useful when angioplasty has failed, resulted in renal artery damage, or there is a solitary functioning kidney. Such manoeuvres may delay the need for dialysis and improve blood pressure control.

PRIMARY ALDOSTERONISM

9.31 What are the causes of primary aldosteronism?

A number of conditions can give rise to primary hyperaldosteronism (*Table 9.1*), which is characterized by excessive aldosterone production beyond that required to maintain electrolyte homeostasis. The most common underlying cause is an aldosterone-producing adrenal adenoma – Conn's syndrome. The pathophysiology of Conn's syndrome remains unknown, although there may be a genetic basis, and it can occur as a component of multiple endocrine neoplasia type I.

The frequency of primary hyperaldosteronism amongst hypertensive subjects is difficult to define, not least because traditionally hypokalaemia was considered to be the best pointer to underlying primary hyperaldosteronism. However, using this selection criterion for further diagnostic investigation appears to significantly underestimate the frequency of hyperaldosteronism. Indeed, widespread screening, and more sensitive investigations suggest that the incidence of primary hyperaldosteronism among hypertensive patients may be as high as 10–15%.

TABLE 9.1 The incidence of primary aldosteronism, classified by underlying pathological diagnosis

Type	Incidence (%)
Aldosterone-producing adenomas	
Classic or angiotensin II unresponsive	57
Angiotensin II responsive	3
Zona glomerulosa hyperplasia	
Bilateral	
Primary adrenal hyperplasia	35
Angiotensin II responsive	5
Unilateral	<1
Aldosterone-producing adrenal carcinoma	<1
Aldosterone-producing extra-adrenal tumours	<1
Glucocorticoid-suppressible aldosteronism	<1

From Irony *et al* 1990, with permission of Elsevier Science.

9.32 What features suggest primary hyperaldosteronism?

Symptoms of primary hyperaldosteronism are generally non-specific but include tiredness, muscle weakness, thirst, polyuria, and nocturia due to hypokalaemia. Hypokalaemia (serum potassium <3.5 mmol/l), or a tendency to hypokalaemia, may be suggestive of underlying primary hyperaldosteronism. However, the majority of patients will have normal serum potassium concentrations, even when an adenoma has been confirmed histologically. It should be remembered that antihypertensive medication, particularly diuretics, could be responsible for hypokalaemia because of their interaction with the renin–angiotensin–aldosterone system. A more reliable screening test may be the ratio of plasma aldosterone to renin. A ratio of >800 makes the diagnosis of primary hyperaldosteronism likely, and warrants further diagnostic investigation. However, drug therapy, e.g. β-blockers or ACE inhibitors, can make interpretation of the ratio difficult.

9.33 How can primary aldosteronism be diagnosed?

Hypokalaemia is insensitive and non-specific, and thus unhelpful in establishing a diagnosis of primary hyperaldosteronism. Random measurement of serum aldosterone concentration is difficult to interpret owing to moment-by-moment fluctuations and an underlying pattern of circadian variation. More useful is measurement of the ratio between plasma aldosterone concentration (pmol/l) and plasma renin activity (pmol/ml/h), where a ratio of <400 is normal; >800 is strongly suggestive of primary aldosteronism due to adenoma. It is important that patients have received no antihypertensive treatment for at least 3 weeks before the tests are performed, which can require careful monitoring in patients with severe hypertension. The diagnosis can be either confirmed by measuring 24-hour urinary aldosterone excretion while patients are adhering to a high-sodium diet, or serum aldosterone level can be measured during administration of intravenous saline, or fludrocortisone, where the diagnosis is indicated by failure to cause significant suppression of circulating concentrations. Alternatively, one can move directly to high-resolution computerized tomography (CT) or MRI scanning of the adrenal glands to distinguish adrenal hyperplasia or adenoma. Because of the high frequency of adrenal 'incidentalomas', venous sampling is often used to prove that a lesion is responsible for excess aldosterone production.

9.34   Which drugs are effective in treating primary aldosteronism?

 An early mechanism by which primary aldosteronism leads to increased blood pressure is through enhanced sodium and water retention, because of its direct effects on the distal renal tubule. With chronicity, the effects of this are partially overcome by the initial rise in blood pressure causing a 'pressure natriuresis', along with upregulation of natriuretic factors. However, blood pressure continues to rise despite achieving fluid volume homeostasis, which may be due to the ability of aldosterone to enhance sensitivity of the peripheral vasculature to constrictor agents, for example angiotensin II and noradrenaline (norepinephrine). Based on these mechanisms, several therapeutic strategies have been used for optimal blood pressure control.

Spironolactone directly antagonizes aldosterone at the mineralocorticoid receptor level and can cause a very marked fall in systemic blood pressure. Historically, dosages of 400–800 mg daily were used, and led to blood pressure reductions of 40–60 mmHg. However, these high dosages were associated with a significant level of adverse effects, for example in one study gynaecomastia was reported in about one-half of patients. In practice, 50–200 mg is usually considered sufficient to achieve satisfactory aldosterone blockade, and in about half of those treated monotherapy allows adequate blood pressure control.

Amiloride and triamterene are epithelial sodium-channel blockers, which also show efficacy by substantially lowering blood pressure in primary hyperaldosteronism. These drugs counter, at least in part, the effects of aldosterone on the renal tubules, and thus prevent excess sodium and water retention. They are useful when spironolactone cannot be tolerated.

Calcium-channel blockers lower blood pressure through effects that are largely independent of the renin–angiotensin–aldosterone system. Calcium is the final common intracellular messenger for several peptide hormones, and it has been suggested that calcium-channel blockers may offer additional benefits in treating hypertension due to primary aldosteronism, perhaps by inhibiting the secretion of aldosterone, or reducing the peripheral vascular response to angiotensin II. However, in practice, there are conflicting reports and calcium-channel blockers do not appear to have any consistent effect on circulating aldosterone concentration, nor do they confer any substantial additional benefit in blood pressure control over that of spironolactone alone.

The contribution of ACE-dependent aldosterone production in primary aldosteronism is not clearly defined. Furthermore, plasma renin activity is already generally suppressed and, therefore, ACE inhibitors are less likely to be effective in the majority of patients. Angiotensin-receptor antagonists are a comparatively novel group of drugs, which could be expected to show greater blood pressure-lowering efficacy than ACE inhibitors because they are able to directly block angiotensin II produced by non-ACE-dependent pathways. Anecdotal reports indicate that these agents can be effective in lowering blood pressure in patients with primary aldosteronism, but their effects in larger patient groups have not yet been demonstrated.

9.35 Which drugs are contraindicated in treatment of primary aldosteronism?

Diuretics, other than potassium-sparing diuretics (*as outlined in Q. 9.34*), should be avoided as monotherapy, because these may aggravate hypokalaemia and increase the risk of arrhythmic death in patients with primary aldosteronism. In unselected hypertensive patients recruited to the SHEP study, the annual occurrence of hypokalaemia (<3.5 mmol/l) was 7.2% among those receiving low-dose thiazide diuretics, compared to 1.0% in those receiving placebo.

It is conceivable that those patients who develop hypokalaemia in response to low-dose thiazide treatment have undiagnosed primary aldosteronism, and it may be useful to institute treatment with spironolactone and assess blood pressure response in these individuals.

9.36 Which patients require adrenalectomy?

The role of surgery will depend on the subtype of primary aldosteronism, and patient comorbidities that may determine suitability. In cases of unilateral adrenal adenoma, resection can potentially lead to a biochemical cure, whereas in bilateral adrenal hyperplasia, medical treatment is indicated. Resolution of hypertension after surgical intervention is less clear-cut, although it improves in the vast majority of patients.

PHAEOCHROMOCYTOMA

9.37 What is a phaeochromocytoma?

A phaeochromocytoma is a catecholamine-secreting tumour of chromaffin cells (*Fig. 9.3*). Some chromaffin cells condense to form the adrenal medulla whereas others remain dispersed, settling adjacent to sympathetic nerves and ganglions. Therefore, phaeochromocytomas can be adrenal or extra-adrenal tumours. Functional tumours of extra-adrenal chromaffin tissue have been referred to as extra-adrenal phaeochromocytomas or functioning paragangliomas. The adrenal medulla normally secretes catecholamines (adrenaline (epinephrine) and noradrenaline (norepinephrine)) into the bloodstream, and functioning tumours of the adrenal medulla (phaeochromocytomas) are among a number of endocrine causes of hypertension. Such tumours not only secrete catecholamines but also have the capacity to synthesize and secrete other biologically active substances, which may account for some of the atypical or anomalous features associated with phaeochromocytoma. However, most of the clinical manifestations of phaeochromocytoma are explicable in terms of excess catecholamine secretion.

Approximately 10% of phaeochromocytomas are extra-adrenal, the majority of these being intra-abdominal. Extra-adrenal phaeochromocytomas exhibit a greater potential for malignancy (30–40%) than tumours of the adrenal gland (3–11%). Phaeochromocytoma has been

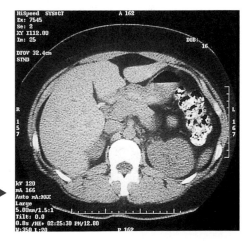

Fig. 9.3 Phaeochromocytoma. A 4 × 5 cm lesion in the left adrenal gland.

associated with a number of familial neuroendocrine symptoms: multiple endocrine neoplasia type IIa (MENIIa) (medullary carcinoma of the thyroid, hyperparathyroidism and phaeochromocytoma), MENIIb (medullary carcinoma of the thyroid, ganglioneuromatosis, hypertrophic corneal nerves and phaeochromocytoma), von Hippel–Lindau disease and neurofibromatosis.

9.38 What is the prevalence/incidence?

The exact prevalence of phaeochromocytoma is uncertain, but population studies suggest that it is very low, and as many as 50% of cases are diagnosed post-mortem. Hypertensive patients account for over 50% of all cases and a prevalence of 0.3% has been reported in a large 50-year autopsy series from the Mayo Clinic, and between 0.1% and 0.5% in two others. Phaeochromocytoma affects men and women equally with a peak incidence during the third and fourth decades of life.

9.39 What features are suggestive of phaeochromocytoma?

SYMPTOMS

Symptoms commonly associated with phaeochromocytoma have been reviewed and are listed in Box 9.6. Most can be attributed to increased levels of circulating catecholamines and there is generally no correlation between symptoms and the size, location or histological appearance of the tumour. An important point to note is that the symptoms are classically paroxysmal, making the condition notoriously difficult to diagnose.

BOX 9.6 Symptoms in patients with phaeochromocytoma in order of decreasing frequency

- Headache
- Sweating
- Palpitations
- Pallor
- Nausea
- Anxiety
- Tremor
- Abdominal pain
- Chest pain
- Weakness
- Visual disturbance
- Dyspnoea
- Weight loss
- Flushing

Most patients with phaeochromocytoma are, however, symptomatic; the most common symptoms being headache, palpitations with or without associated tachycardia and excessive inappropriate sweating. The occurrence of this triad in a hypertensive patient is highly suggestive of phaeochromocytoma, whereas lack of all these symptoms makes the diagnosis unlikely but not impossible. Flushing is so uncommon in phaeochromocytoma as to cast serious doubt on the diagnosis, but can rarely occur due to co-secretion of a vasodilator peptide such as calcitonin-gene-related peptide CGRP.

SIGNS

The only persisting abnormal physical signs relate to blood pressure. The majority of patients exhibit sustained hypertension, although wild fluctuations in blood pressure are characteristic even in patients with background hypertension. Paroxysmal episodes of hypertension may occur spontaneously or be precipitated by exercise, palpation of the tumour, defecation or drug administration, including antidepressants, phenothiazines, metoclopramide or β-blockers.

9.40 How should patients be investigated?

Once the clinical suspicion of phaeochromocytoma has been raised, the diagnosis must be supported by evidence of excessive catecholamine secretion. In the first instance this depends on demonstration of increased urinary excretion of catecholamines or their metabolites. Criteria for biochemical screening should be hypertensive patients with the additional features listed in Box 9.6. This accepts that there will inevitably be a fraction of false positives.

In patients with biochemical evidence of phaeochromocytoma, the next step is to distinguish patients with hypertension and sympathetic overactivity from patients with a phaeochromocytoma. Diagnostic accuracy has been improved by the development of tests designed to suppress catecholamine levels in patients without phaeochromocytoma. Brown and colleagues pioneered the use of the autonomic ganglion blocker pentolinium in this respect. In subjects with sympathetic overactivity, pentolinium suppresses levels of adrenaline (epinephrine) and noradrenaline (norepinephrine), but does not suppress catecholamine levels in subjects with phaeochromocytoma (Brown *et al* 1981). Pentolinium is rarely used now and has been replaced by the clonidine suppression test. Clonidine is an α_2-receptor agonist which decreases sympathetic outflow and thus suppresses sympathetic overactivity without influencing catecholamine secretion by a phaeochromocytoma.

Once diagnosed biochemically, the next step is to localize the tumour. Abdominal ultrasound and CT scanning are helpful in this respect, although 10% of phaeochromocytomas are extra-adrenal and some of these may be extra-abdominal. Tumours secreting mainly noradrenaline are more likely to be extra-adrenal owing to the fact that the enzymatic step to convert noradrenaline to adrenaline is usually absent in extra-adrenal tumours.

Finally, an adrenal or extra-adrenal mass may not necessarily be a functioning phaeochromocytoma, and scanning with metaiodobenzylguanidine (MIBG) allows visualization of functioning adrenal or extra-adrenal chromaffin tissue with a reported specificity of 98% and a sensitivity in excess of 80% (*Fig. 9.4*).

9.41 How should a hypertensive crisis be managed?

A hypertensive crisis associated with phaeochromocytoma is a life-threatening condition and should be managed acutely with intravenous administration of an α-blocker such as phentolamine. A good response to phentolamine in an unexplained hypertensive crisis should raise the suspicion of a phaeochromocytoma. Following initial intravenous phentolamine, oral therapy with an irreversible α-blocker such as phenoxybenzamine should be used. β-blockade should not be used in the situation of a hypertensive crisis, as this would lead to unopposed stimulation of α-receptors by the uncontrolled catecholamine levels and may exacerbate the hypertension.

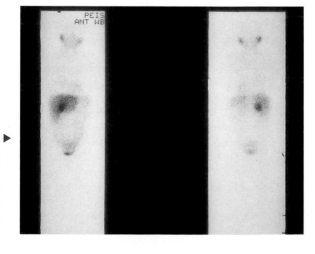

Fig. 9.4 A radio-isotope scan with MIBG, showing localization of tracer to the left adrenal, confirming the solitary nature of the tumour.

9.42   Are β-blockers contraindicated?

Although β-blockers are not absolutely contraindicated, they should not be used without concomitant α-blockade. This is because unopposed α-stimulation by adrenaline (epinephrine) and noradrenaline (norepinephrine) may cause vasoconstriction and a paradoxical rise in blood pressure. Once a patient has been adequately α-blocked with phenoxybenzamine, it is often necessary to introduce β-blockade to suppress the reflex tachycardia due to the phenoxybenzamine.

9.43   What drugs can be used to control blood pressure?

The cornerstone of drug therapy to control blood pressure in phaeochromocytoma is α-adrenoceptor blockade. The drug of choice is the irreversible α-blocker phenoxybenzamine. This acetylating agent forms a stable covalent bond with the α-receptor. It is introduced at low doses (10 mg b.d.) and the dose titrated upwards until blood pressure is controlled. During this time, additional doses of a reversible α-blocker, intravenous phentolamine or oral prazosin or doxazosin, depending on the degree of urgency, can be used to control spikes of blood pressure. When the patient begins to experience side-effects from α-blockade – postural hypotension, dry mouth and sedation – this is taken as evidence of adequate α-blockade. Since phenoxybenzamine also blocks presynaptic α_2-receptors, the usual feedback loop at sympathetic nerve terminals is blocked, and patients often experience troublesome tachycardia. At this stage β-blockade can be safely introduced to counteract this effect and provide further blood pressure control.

9.44   What are the indications for surgery?

Benign phaeochromocytomas should always be surgically removed if this is safely possible. This is because, whilst they are present, the patient is always at risk of a fatal hypertensive crisis. In addition, symptoms are extremely distressing to the patient. Surgical removal should only normally be attempted as an elective procedure with the patient being admitted to hospital preoperatively for appropriate preparation, and should involve a multidisciplinary team comprising an endocrine surgeon, an experienced anaesthetist and a clinical pharmacologist as well as an intensive care specialist. Specialized nursing should also be available.

Occasionally phaeochromocytomas are malignant and multiple, making surgical removal impossible. Malignant phaeochromocytomas are uncommon, accounting for 10–12% of all cases. No clinical feature is absolutely diagnostic of malignancy although extra-adrenal tumours exhibit a greater potential for malignancy (30–40%) and also tumours that secrete dopamine rather than adrenaline (epinephrine) and noradrenaline (norepinephrine). In this setting, inhibition of catecholamine biosynthesis by α-methyl-P-tyrosine may be useful. Experience with cytotoxic therapy is limited but survival rates of 56% have been reported with a combination of cyclophosphamide, vincristine and decarbazine. [131]I MIBG has also been used to target chemotherapy to functioning phaeochromocytoma tissue, with encouraging results.

9.45 How should patients be prepared for surgery?

 Surgery should always be performed as an elective procedure with patients admitted to hospital for adequate preparation. Subjects should be α-blocked with oral phenoxybenzamine until they become symptomatic (postural hypotension, dry mouth, drowsiness). Because of chronic exposure to catecholamines, patients are often volume-deplete and this should be adequately corrected preoperatively. Daily weighing is helpful in this respect and it is always best to err on the side of caution, and delay surgery if there is any doubt as to the volume status.

PREMEDICATION

Droperidol inhibits catecholamine uptake and is therefore contraindicated, as are phenothiazines. Morphine and atropine may both cause release of catecholamines and are, therefore, also contraindicated. If an anticholinergic is required hyoscine is an acceptable alternative.

PEROPERATIVE MEDICATION

Following removal of the tumour, the major concern is sudden and severe hypotension. This is minimized by α-blockade and volume expansion preoperatively. If arterial pressure fails to respond to i.v. fluids, a pressor agent is required. However, drugs acting as catecholamine receptors (adrenaline (epinephrine), noradrenaline (norepinephrine), dopamine and dobutamine) are unlikely to be effective because of α-blockade and receptor downregulation due to chronic exposure to catecholamines. Angiotensin II is therefore preferred and is given by i.v. infusion at a rate of 1–2 ng/kg/min increasing as necessary to 10 mg/kg/min. Angiotensin II infusion should be available pre-prepared as severe hypotension is an emergency situation.

CUSHING'S SYNDROME

9.46 How can Cushing's syndrome be classified?

The causes of Cushing's syndrome may be broadly classified into two groups:

- ACTH-dependent, in which steroid overproduction is secondary to inappropriately high ACTH levels

■ ACTH-independent, in which the steroid production is autonomous and leads to suppression of ACTH levels (*Box 9.7*).

BOX 9.7 Causes of Cushing's disease

ACTH-dependent
■ Pituitary-dependent Cushing's syndrome (Cushing's disease)
■ Ectopic ACTH production (e.g. oat cell carcinoma)
■ Ectopic CRH production

ACTH-independent
■ Adrenal adenoma
■ Adrenal carcinoma
■ Multinodular adrenal hyperplasia
■ Exogenous steroid administration

9.47 What are the symptoms and signs of Cushing's syndrome?

With the exception of the increased pigmentation seen in patients with ACTH-secreting tumours (due to the sequence homology between ACTH and MSH), all the features of Cushing's syndrome depend directly on steroid overproduction.

The clinical features seen in a particular patient are therefore dependent on the type of steroid overproduced and the rate of onset of the condition, but can be broadly classified into physical and metabolic features (*Box 9.8*). Again the speed of onset will determine whether physical or metabolic features predominate in any one patient.

9.48 How should patients be investigated?

As the onset of Cushing's syndrome may be insidious, it is important to consider the diagnosis in patients who present with hypertension, diabetes, proximal myopathy, hirsutism or osteoporosis, particularly if more than one of these features is present and associated with hypertension. Investigation of patients with suspected Cushing's syndrome involves screening tests to distinguish between Cushing's syndrome and patients with obesity, hypertension or diabetes. Then definitive tests are needed to establish the diagnosis of Cushing's syndrome, and finally tests are aimed at defining the underlying cause of the condition.

SCREENING TESTS

Screening can be achieved by either using an overnight dexamethasone suppression test or measurement of 24-hour urinary free cortisol excretion. Providing an accurate, reliable 24-hour urine collection can be achieved, free cortisol excretion is a simple, sensitive and specific means of

---

BOX 9.8 Features of Cushing's disease

Physical

- Central obesity   >90%
- Myopathy   60%
- Striae   50%
- Hypertension   70%
- Hirsutism/acne   80%
- Amenorrhoea   80%
- Back pain   60%
- Psychological disturbance 40%
- Diabetes/glucose intolerance 10%

Metabolic

- Hyperinsulinaemia
- Insulin resistance
- Increased proteolysis
- Decreased collagen synthesis
- Poor wound healing
- Depressed immune system and increased rise of infections
  $\downarrow$ cellular immunity
- Lymphopenia
- Osteoporosis
- $\uparrow$ circulating PTH

---

establishing the diagnosis. Normally, only 1% of cortisol from the adrenals is secreted unchanged in the urine, and when circulating cortisol levels are increased, as in Cushing's syndrome, this fraction increases disproportionately. Although normal ranges of free cortisol vary between laboratories, the upper limit of normal is around 100 μg/day. In normal subjects, administration of dexamethasone (1 mg) will suppress the adrenal axis with no interference with cortisol measurements. In patients with suspected Cushing's syndrome, 1 mg of dexamethasone can be administered at 11.00 p.m. and plasma cortisol is then measured at 8.00 a.m. the next day. In patients with Cushing's, little or no suppression is seen and cortisol levels remain >10 μg/dl. False negative results are rare, but false positives may occur in patients with concomitant non-specific illness.

Further investigations to confirm the diagnosis and establish the cause include midnight cortisol levels (to demonstrate disruption of the normal diurnal cortisol excretion rhythm in patients with Cushing's syndrome); low- and high-dose dexamethasone suppression tests; plasma ACTH; and imaging of the pituitary and adrenal gland. Excess alcohol intake and anorexia nervosa may have similar biochemical features to Cushing's syndrome and should, therefore, be excluded.

9.49 What are the principles of management?

The management of Cushing's syndrome is critically dependent on the underlying cause, as outlined previously. The principal aim should be to cure the patient without inducing any iatrogenic deficiency states.

ADRENAL TUMOURS

The treatment of an adrenal adenoma is unilateral adrenalectomy. Results from this operation are usually excellent. However, it should be remembered that due to suppression of the hyperthalamo-pituitary axis and the contralateral adrenal gland, there is a risk of postoperative adrenal insufficiency. Steroid cover is, therefore, given peri- and postoperatively.

ADRENAL CARCINOMA

The prognosis for patients with adrenal carcinoma is poor. Metastases are often present at the time of diagnosis (most usually to the liver and lungs) and the median survival is around 4 years. Surgery is the treatment of choice to reduce tumour bulk. Drug treatment for metastatic or residual tumour is mitotone, a drug which reduces secretion of cortisol in around 70% of patients. However, use of mitotone is often limited by its side-effects. Adrenal carcinomas are not usually radiosensitive, although chemotherapy with cisplatin has been used.

ACTH-SECRETING TUMOURS

Where possible, the treatment of Cushing's syndrome due to ectopic ACTH-secreting tumours is resection of the primary tumour. Results of surgery are, however, usually poor especially if the primary tumour is carcinoma of the bronchus. The results of resection of a carcinoid tumour are usually much better. Therefore, the major aim of therapy in such patients is to minimize metabolic disturbance and improve the quality of life. To this end, a number of therapeutic options are available. Metyrapone inhibits 11β-hydroxylase and inhibits cortisol biosynthesis. Alternatively, ketoconazole will also inhibit steroid biosynthesis. Finally, aminoglutethimide can also be used to block steroid synthesis.

CUSHING'S DISEASE (PITUITARY OVERSECRETION OF ACTH)

Originally Cushing's disease was treated by bilateral adrenalectomy. However, this operation, although effective, was highly problematical. There is an operative mortality of between 5–10%, a high incidence of postoperative complications and a significant recurrence rate. In addition, patients are permanently dependent on glucocorticoid and mineralocorticoid replacement therapy. Moreover, the bilateral adrenalectomy often results in Nelson's syndrome (a condition associated with excessive skin pigmentation). This is due to the fact that ACTH levels increase post-surgery and ACTH has considerable sequence homology with melanin-stimulating hormone (MSH). Therefore, pituitary surgery has become the treatment of choice. In patients with microadenomas, the results are excellent and there is a cure in approximately 85% of patients. In the minority of patients with a macroadenoma, results are much worse, with only 25% achieving a cure. Second-line treatment includes radiotherapy, which although effective in children, is much less so in adults. Insertion of radioactive yttrium in the sella has been used, resulting in remission in around 65% of patients.

Finally, drug therapy with enzyme inhibitors to block steroid production has been used, although results are not as good as when used in the treatment of ectopic ACTH production.

9.50 What are the indications for surgery?

As discussed above (Q. 9.49), surgery is the preferred option for the treatment of Cushing's syndrome irrespective of its aetiology. The results of surgery are best in adrenal adenomas and patients with ectopic ACTH production from a carcinoid tumour.

COARCTATION OF THE AORTA

9.51 What is coarctation?

Coarctation is a congenital narrowing of the aorta, which may be a localized band or more diffuse narrowing. It may occur anywhere in the aorta, but usually is located just distal to the origin of the left subclavian artery or distal to the insertion of the ligamentum arteriosum. It is associated with bicuspid aortic valves (50% of cases), and cerebral aneurysms. The prevalence is ~1:10 000, and it is more common in males (2:1). It can be associated with other conditions such as Turner's syndrome.

9.52 Is it only found in children?

Most cases of coarctation are diagnosed in childhood. However, 20% of cases are identified in adolescents and adults. It may present with heart failure in infancy or incidental hypertension in young adults.

9.53 What are the typical features of coarctation?

The classical findings in coarctation are upper body hypertension, weak femoral pulses, and radiofemoral delay. In addition there is usually a widespread systolic murmur heard over the coarctation, especially in the back. Occasionally, this may be continuous if the coarctation is severe. There may also be a forceful apex beat due to left ventricular hypertrophy, an aortic systolic murmur due to the presence of a bicuspid aortic valve, and rib-notching visible on the chest X-ray. An ECG is likely to show left ventricular hypertrophy. Rarely, coarctation may present with malignant hypertension.

9.54 How should the diagnosis be confirmed?

CT or MRI angiography can be used to confirm the diagnosis. The coarctation can also be identified by echocardiography, which may also be used to assess pressure gradients, and to check the aortic value.

9.55 What is the treatment of choice?

Surgical correction, usually in childhood, is the treatment of choice. Recurrence rates are lower if the procedure is not performed in infancy, but if delayed until after the age of 7 there is an increased risk of long-term hypertension. Repair substantially improves survival, but life-expectancy is still below normal. Moreover, a proportion of patients (~20%) remain hypertensive post-surgery, requiring life-long antihypertensive therapy. The reasons for this are unknown and may reflect largely irreversible structural and neurohormonal adaptations. The role of balloon angioplasty is not yet fully established for primary therapy, but it is used for recurrence post-surgery.

9.56 Can coarctation recur?

Yes. The frequency of recurrence is ~15–30% if the repair is performed in the first year of life, and <10% if undertaken later in childhood.

OTHER SECONDARY CAUSES?

9.57 What is glucocorticoid remediable hypertension?

Also known as glucocorticoid-suppressible hyperaldosteronism, this is an autosomal dominant condition characterized by low-renin hypertension and aldosterone excess. There is disruption of the normal renin–angiotensin–aldosterone system, such that aldosterone secretion is stimulated by corticotrophin (ACTH), which in turn is not sensitive to circulating aldosterone concentrations (Sutherland *et al* 1966). Thus, there is loss of negative feedback and excess aldosterone production. Administration of glucocorticoid, for example dexamethasone, decreases corticotrophin production and, therefore, suppresses aldosterone secretion. There is an International Register for cases, which at present are fewer than 200 in number.

9.58 What is Liddle's syndrome?

This was originally described in a family in which the siblings were affected by early-onset hypertension and hypokalaemia, associated with low circulating renin and aldosterone concentrations (Liddle *et al* 1966). It is due to a mutation of the mineralocorticoid-dependent epithelial sodium channel, which results in constitutive channel activation, even in the absence of mineralocorticoid. Liddle's syndrome is inherited in an autosomal dominant manner, and fails to respond to spironolactone (aldosterone antagonist), but does respond to triamterene (epithelial sodium-channel blocker).

9.59 What is the syndrome of apparent mineralocorticoid excess?

In this syndrome, the concentrations of renin and aldosterone are characteristically low, and cortisol (a glucocorticoid) acts as a potent mineralocorticoid at the mineralocorticoid receptor (Stewart *et al* 1988). The disorder is inherited in an autosomal recessive manner, and has clinical features resembling primary hyperaldosteronism. It can be distinguished by low aldosterone and renin concentrations, and is diagnosed by 24-hour urinary cortisol measurement. Treatment includes spironolactone and amiloride, generally in higher doses than those used to treat primary aldosteronism. Dexamethasone can also be used to suppress endogenous secretion of cortisol.

9.60 Is thyrotoxicosis associated with hypertension?

Cardiovascular manifestations are a frequent finding in hyperthyroid and hypothyroid states, and a number of mechanisms have been proposed to account for how thyroid hormones may exert effects on the cardiovascular system. There is increasing evidence that thyroid hormones exert direct effects on the myocardium, mediated by specific nuclear receptors, which lead to increased messenger RNA production. Thyroid hormones also interact with the sympathetic nervous system so that there is greater responsiveness to sympathetic stimulation. Hyperthyroidism generally has little or no effect on mean arterial blood pressure, although systolic blood pressure is often elevated, and there is an association with tachycardia and atrial tachyarrhythmias. These changes are thought to be mediated by sympathetic activation, and may resolve after medical or surgical correction. There is also increasing evidence for long-term morbidity and mortality associated with thyroid dysfunction, including increased likelihood of cardiovascular and cerebrovascular mortality in subjects with previously treated thyrotoxicosis. Thyroid function tests should be performed where there are clinical features suggesting hyperthyroidism.

9.61   Are there any explanations for severe hypertension in pregnancy

A mutation in the mineralocorticoid receptor that causes early-onset hypertension, markedly exacerbated in pregnancy, has been described (Geller *et al* 2000). This mutation results in constitutive mineralocorticoid receptor activation and alters receptor specificity, such that progesterone and other steroids lacking 21-hydroxyl groups, which are normally receptor antagonists, becoming potent agonists. The structural receptor defect has been characterized and demonstrates the ability of a single amino acid substitution to dramatically alter the consequences of receptor–ligand interaction. Mineralocorticoid receptor mutation represents a new Mendelian form of hypertension with marked exacerbation in pregnancy. This has raised the possibility that other forms of receptor mutation could explain hypertension in a wider context, or the aberrant response to a normal pregnancy-related hormone in pre-eclampsia. Males with the mineralocorticoid receptor mutation also show elevated blood pressure despite low circulating progesterone concentrations, which suggests that constitutive receptor activation may be sufficient to cause hypertension, or that another steroid acts as an agonist at the mutated receptor. However, the described mutation is exceedingly rare and cannot explain the majority of cases of hypertension in pregnancy.

Type 2 diabetes and hypertension

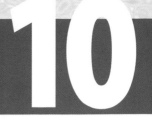

10

EPIDEMIOLOGY AND AETIOLOGY

10.1 Is diabetes a benign condition?

Despite the fact that type 2 diabetes is increasingly common, many clinicians continue to view it as essentially an endocrine disease characterized by hyperglycaemia, and until recently the clinical focus has been on tight glycaemic control. Moreover, type 2 diabetes has tended to be regarded as a 'mild' form of diabetes and essentially benign, especially by the general public and even some clinicians. However, many of the complications seen in type 1 diabetes are increasing in prevalence in patients with type 2 diabetes, including renal failure, blindness and limb amputation. Indeed, the risk of cardiovascular disease is greater in type 2 diabetes than in subjects with type 1. Type 2 diabetes can, therefore, no longer be viewed as benign and should be treated as a vascular disease carrying an unacceptably high risk of heart attack and stroke. This is supported by recent data demonstrating that the mortality from coronary heart disease in patients with type 2 diabetes, who have not had a myocardial infarction, is the same as in non-diabetics post-myocardial infarction (*Fig. 5.1*) (Haffner *et al* 1998). Thus in clinical practice patients with type 2 diabetes should be managed as aggressively as non-diabetics are post-myocardial infarction.

10.2 What is the prevalence of hypertension in diabetes?

The prevalence of hypertension in subjects with type 2 diabetes will, to some extent, be dependent on the definition of hypertension. Using the definition of SBP ≥160 mmHg DBP ≥95 mmHg, the prevalence of hypertension in type 2 diabetes in subjects ≥55 years is 43% in men and 52% in women (Hypertension in Diabetes Study 1993). In the UK Prospective Diabetes Study (UKPDS) the prevalence of hypertension in newly diagnosed type 2 diabetics was 39%. If the criteria of ≥140 and/or ≥90 mmHg are used, ~80% of diabetics are hypertensive in some series.

10.3 Why is hypertension so common in diabetics?

The age-related rise in blood pressure is exaggerated in patients with type 2 diabetes, which is a reflection of the premature vascular ageing associated with this condition that leads to increased arterial stiffening. Such changes account for the fact that isolated systolic hypertension (ISH) is particularly common in patients with type 2 diabetes. Type 2 diabetics are usually insulin resistant and insulin has recently been shown to decrease large artery stiffness, an effect that is blunted in obese insulin-resistant subjects. In addition, there are a number of other mechanisms accounting for the increased incidence of hypertension in type 2 diabetes, and these include diabetic nephropathy and obesity, which are also common in type 2 diabetes. Indeed, the development of microalbuminuria is particularly associated with the development of hypertension. The levels of exchangeable sodium are also increased in type 2 diabetes and are positively correlated with blood pressure. A number of endocrine causes of hypertension may also coexist with diabetes, including thyrotoxicosis, Cushing's syndrome, phaeochromocytoma and acromegaly. Finally, the possibility of a secondary cause of hypertension should always be considered in subjects with diabetes, especially renal artery stenosis.

10.4 What is syndrome X?

It remains unclear as to why individuals with type 2 diabetes have such a high incidence of cardiovascular disease. It has been suggested that it may be due to clustering of additional risk factors in such patients. Common additional risk factors are hypertension, insulin resistance, dyslipidaemia and obesity, which together have been termed *syndrome X*.

10.5 Is secondary hypertension more common in diabetics?

Secondary hypertension is relatively more common amongst type 2 diabetics. Indeed, renal artery stenosis is more common in these patients. Diabetics are also more likely to suffer from thyrotoxicosis, Cushing's syndrome, phaeochromocytoma or acromegaly than non-diabetics, and these conditions can all give rise to hypertension in a proportion of affected individuals.

INVESTIGATION AND TREATMENT

10.6 How often should diabetics have their blood pressure checked?

As previously outlined (Q. *10.2*), the prevalence of hypertension in type 2 diabetes ranges from 39–80% depending on the criteria used. Recent data from the UKPDS clearly show the benefits of tight blood pressure control in newly diagnosed type 2 diabetics. Therefore, all type 2 diabetic patients should have their blood pressure checked at each clinic visit and at least annually if they are well controlled. If control is poor, they should be assessed more frequently (every 3–4 months) until blood pressure is controlled. At least two separate readings should be taken at each visit.

10.7 What level of blood pressure should be treated?

The latest British Hypertension Society guidelines (Ramsay *et al* 1999) recommend that antihypertensive therapy is initiated in patients with type 2 diabetes if blood pressure is sustained at systolic blood pressure ≥160 mmHg and/or diastolic pressure ≥90 mmHg. If the systolic pressure is 140–160 mmHg, then therapy should be initiated if there is microvascular or end-organ damage, or if the risk of coronary heart disease is >15% over 10 years. The optimal blood pressure targets are systolic pressure <130 mmHg and diastolic pressure <80 mmHg. The minimum acceptable level of control (Audit Standard) is systolic blood pressure <140 mmHg and diastolic pressure <90 mmHg. The guidelines do, however, concede that despite best practice, these levels would be difficult to achieve in some individuals with diabetes and hypertension. Indeed, in the UKPDS many subjects with type 2 diabetes required at least triple therapy to achieve adequate blood pressure control.

10.8 What are the benefits of treatment?

The benefits of treating blood pressure in type 2 diabetics have been reported by the UKPDS and are illustrated in Table 10.1.

10.9 Do diabetics benefit more or less from blood pressure lowering?

Subjects with type 2 diabetes are at greater risk of a cardiovascular event than non-diabetics and thus will obtain a greater absolute risk reduction even if antihypertensive therapy produces the same relative reduction as it does in non-diabetic subjects. Indeed, the 583 subjects with type 2 diabetes in the SHEP study obtained twice the absolute risk reduction in cardiovascular events compared to the non-diabetic subjects. Moreover, in the SystEur study there was a greater relative risk reduction in the 492 diabetic subjects treated with a long-acting calcium-channel blocker compared with non-diabetics. Thus diabetics stand to gain at least as much, and probably more, from antihypertensive therapy than do non-diabetics.

TABLE 10.1 Benefits of treating hypertension in type 2 diabetics

	Glycaemic control*	Blood pressure control*
Any diabetes endpoint	20	6
Diabetes-related deaths	91[†]	15
Myocardial infarction	37[†]	20[†]
Stroke	167[†]	20

* Number needed to treat to prevent 1 event.
[†] Not significant.
Data from the UKPDS.

10.10 Does blood pressure reduction reduce microvascular complications?

Data from the UKPDS show that tight blood pressure control in a cohort of newly diagnosed subjects with type 2 diabetes is effective in reducing microvascular complications (UK Prospective Diabetes Study Group 1998a). Indeed, tight blood pressure control was more effective at preventing diabetic retinopathy than tight blood glucose control, a finding that was surprising, and is as yet not fully explained.

10.11 Does blood pressure reduction reduce macrovascular complications?

Again the UKPDS showed that neither tight blood pressure control nor tight glycaemic control significantly reduces the incidence of myocardial infarction (*Table 10.1*) (UK Prospective Diabetes Study Group 1998a, b). However, although tight glycaemic control had no effect on stroke, tight blood pressure control reduced the incidence of stroke by 44%. Moreover, other large studies, which included type 2 diabetic subjects, have clearly shown a reduction in cardiovascular events following tight blood pressure control (*Q. 10.9*), and since they are at higher risk, the absolute reduction in macrovascular events would be greater in subjects with diabetes than in non-diabetics.

10.12 Does blood pressure reduction benefit diabetic nephropathy?

There is overwhelming evidence that blood pressure reduction will slow the progression of diabetic nephropathy. In addition, there is evidence to suggests that ACE inhibitors are of greater benefit than other antihypertensive agents (Agardh *et al* 1996, Cooper 1998). For this reason, subjects with diabetic nephropathy should be treated with ACE inhibition unless there is an absolute contraindication such as renal artery stenosis. Nevertheless, since renal artery stenosis is more common in subjects with type 2 diabetes, ACE inhibition should be introduced with caution, and urea and electrolytes checked after initiation of therapy. More recently, two studies have demonstrated that angiotensin II receptor antagonists ('sartans') slow the progression of renal disease in type 2 diabetics (*Q. 7.38*).

10.13 Do elderly diabetics benefit less from treatment?

All the evidence suggests that elderly diabetics benefit more from treatment. This is because elderly diabetics are at increased risk compared to younger subjects with diabetes. Furthermore, the largest reductions in cardiovascular events have been seen in the elderly diabetic population treated in the SystEur study (*Q. 10.9*).

10.14 Which drug should be used in patients with type 2 diabetes?

The major objective in treating hypertension in patients with type 2 diabetes is tight blood pressure control. Indeed, the British Hypertension Society target blood pressure for diabetics with hypertension is lower than that for non-diabetics (Ramsay *et al* 1999). No class of antihypertensive agent is absolutely contraindicated and the UKPDS showed no difference in outcome between those treated with an ACE inhibitor and those receiving a β-blocker. To date, trial evidence would suggest that, especially in elderly diabetics, diuretic and calcium-channel blocker regimes are highly effective in reducing cardiovascular events. In patients with diabetic nephropathy, ACE inhibition is strongly indicated to slow the progression of the renal condition (*Q. 10.12*). In diabetic patients with hypertension and previous myocardial infarction, ACE inhibitors and β-blockers would be particularly indicated, as indeed they are in non-diabetic subjects following myocardial infarction.

10.15 Are diuretics contraindicated?

Although many still believe that diuretics are contraindicated in type 2 diabetes, this is not supported by trial evidence. Indeed, the diabetics included in the SHEP study, which had a treatment regime based on thiazide diuretics, received substantially more benefit than non-diabetics in terms of cardiovascular risk reduction (*Q. 10.9*).

10.16 Are β-blockers contraindicated?

No, although it has been suggested that β-blockers may have adverse effects in subjects with type 2 diabetes. The UKPDS showed them to be equally effective at reducing cardiovascular events as ACE inhibition.

10.17 Should ACE inhibitors be used first-line?

Again, with the exception of patients with diabetic nephropathy, there is little evidence to support the use of ACE inhibitors as first-line therapy. Both diuretic and calcium-channel blocker regimes have been shown to be effective, especially in more elderly subjects with diabetes, and the major goal of therapy is to achieve adequate blood pressure reduction irrespective of the drug used. However, many patients with type 2 diabetes do require two or three agents in combination to achieve adequate blood pressure control.

10.18 Do ACE inhibitors increase the risk of hyperglycaemia?

There is no evidence that ACE inhibition increases the risk of hyperglycaemia. Indeed, as ACE inhibition has been shown to improve insulin sensitivity, the theoretical risk is of hypoglycaemia. However, although a number of small studies have demonstrated that hypoglycaemia is associated with ACE inhibition, this was not supported by data from the UKPDS using captopril.

10.19 Does anti-hypertensive treatment prevent diabetes?

There is no direct trial evidence that antihypertensive therapy prevents the onset of diabetes. However, subgroup analysis of larger studies has suggested that ACE inhibition may reduce the incidence of diabetes (HOPE and CAPP studies). However, statin therapy has also been shown to have a similar effect, and thus any possible mechanism is unclear. Large properly controlled and randomized trials will be necessary to address this important question in the future.

10.20 Do antihypertensive drugs interact with oral hypoglycaemics?

There is no evidence to contraindicate the use of any class of antihypertensive agent in type 2 diabetics treated with oral hyperglycaemic agents. This is fortunate because, as previously stated, many subjects with type 2 diabetes will require triple therapy to achieve adequate blood pressure control.

10.21 Does tight glycaemic control decrease blood pressure?

As yet, there is no evidence that tight glycaemic control lowers blood pressure. However, given the fact that insulin can decrease arterial stiffness and tight glycaemic control decreases insulin resistance, it may be that better glycaemic control may lower central aortic blood pressure. This possibility will need further investigation in the future as many patients with type 2 diabetes also have isolated systolic hypertension. Interestingly, cholesterol reduction with statin therapy has indeed been shown to lower blood pressure, although not in a diabetic population. As a number of studies involving cholesterol reduction in type 2 diabetic subjects are ongoing, it may be that a similar blood pressure reduction with statin therapy in type 2 diabetics will be demonstrated.

Hypertension in the elderly

11

EPIDEMIOLOGY AND AETIOLOGY

11.1 What happens to blood pressure with age?

Systolic blood pressure increases continuously throughout adult life. In contrast, diastolic pressure rises until the age of 50 years, then plateaus and, after the age of 60 years, actually then decreases (Franklin *et al* 1997). Therefore, pulse pressure (systolic – diastolic) widens with age (*Fig. 11.1*), whereas mean arterial pressure changes by much less. This trend is observed in almost all populations world-wide.

11.2 What is the incidence of hypertension in the elderly?

Hypertension in the elderly is very common. Indeed, it affects more than half of the over 60s if ≥160/100 mmHg is used as a definition, and more than 70% if the JNC VI (USA) criteria of ≥140/90 mmHg are employed (Primatesta *et al* 2001).

11.3 What is the most common form of hypertension in the elderly?

Isolated systolic hypertension is by far the most common form of hypertension in the elderly (*Fig. 1.1*). It affects around 25% of elderly hypertensive subjects (≥160 and <90 mmHg), or 50% if the JNC VI criteria are used (≥140 and <90 mmHg) (Wilking *et al* 1988, Franklin *et al* 2001, Primatesta *et al* 2001).

11.4 Is elevated systolic blood pressure in older subjects benign?

Although systolic hypertension in the elderly was for many years considered benign, a wealth of data show this to be completely untrue (Nielsen *et al* 1995). Indeed, isolated systolic hypertension is associated with considerable excess cardiovascular morbidity and mortality; it increases the risk of stroke by around 60%, and of coronary disease by around 40%.

11.5 What are the risks of hypertension in the elderly?

Hypertension in the elderly is a potent risk factor for cerebrovascular and coronary artery disease, and the development of heart failure (Sagie *et al* 1993, Nielsen *et al* 1995, O'Donnell *et al* 1997). Antihypertensive therapy for both essential hypertension and isolated systolic hypertension in the elderly is effective in reducing the incidence of these complications (Mulrow *et al* 2000).

INVESTIGATION AND TREATMENT

11.6 Is automated sphygmomanometry reliable in older subjects?

Oscillometric sphygmomanometers may be unreliable in older subjects with

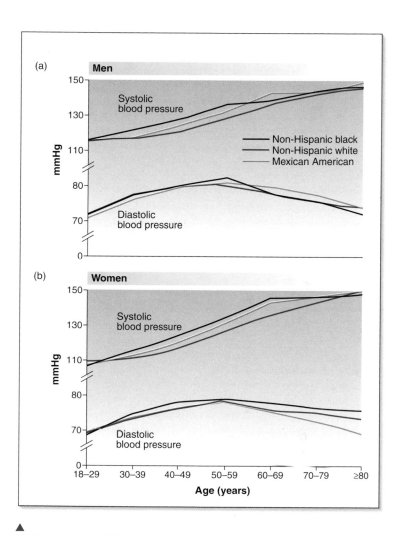

Fig. 11.1 Age-related changes in blood pressure. Mean systolic and diastolic blood pressure by age, gender and race, in a US population. (From Burt VL, Whelton P, Roccella EJ *et al* 1995 Prevalence of hypertension in the US adult population. Results from the Third National Health and Nutrition Examination Survey, 1988–1991. Hypertension 25:305–313, with permission of Lippincott, Williams & Wilkins.)

stiffened arteries (van Popele *et al* 2000). Indeed, many of the algorithms that oscillometric devices employ are based on work in younger subjects. Similarly, validation of these instruments is often conducted in young people rather than elderly hypertensives. Therefore, if in doubt check the blood pressure with a calibrated mercury sphygmomanometer.

11.7 How often should the elderly be screened for hypertension?

Current guidelines recommend that blood pressure be assessed every 5 years in all adults, but annually if the blood pressure is >135/85 mmHg. Given the very high prevalence of hypertension and borderline hypertension in the elderly, annual assessment of blood pressure is required in the majority of adults over 60.

11.8 Should hypertension in the elderly be treated?

Yes. The benefits of treating hypertension in the elderly have been well documented (*see Table 11.1*). This applies to both elevated systolic and/or diastolic pressure (*Fig. 11.2*) and systolic pressure in isolation (*Fig. 11.3*). Moreover, the relative benefit from treatment in older subjects is at least the same, if not greater, than that observed in younger individuals. Therefore, since the elderly are at higher risk of cardiovascular disease, they stand to obtain a greater absolute risk reduction.

11.9 What level of blood pressure should be treated?

The available evidence suggests that all subjects with sustained blood pressure >160/100 mmHg should be treated, and this should be the first priority. Individuals with pressures >140/90 mmHg should receive therapy if their risk of coronary heart disease is >15% per annum, or there is evidence of end-organ damage, which includes coronary or cerebrovascular disease. This applies to patients with both essential hypertension and isolated systolic hypertension. Despite the clear evidence supporting these recommendations, data from the UK and USA suggest that physicians have a bias against treating the elderly hypertensive (Dickerson & Brown 1995, Franklin *et al* 2001).

TABLE 11.1 Benefits of antihypertensive therapy in the elderly

Outcome measure	% reduction	NNT*
Cardiovascular morbidity and mortality	5.2	19
Cardiovascular mortality	2.0	50
Total mortality	1.7	63

* Number needed to treat (*see Q. 5.6*).
Source: Mulrow *et al* (2000).

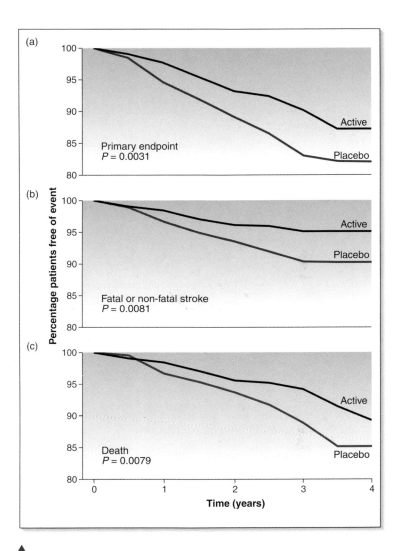

Fig. 11.2 Effect of antihypertensive treatment in older hypertensives. Results of the STOP trial in 70- to 84-year-olds treated with thiazides and β-blockers or placebo. (From Dahlof *et al* 1991, with permission of Elsevier Science.)

11.10 What are the targets to aim for?

The British Hypertension Society suggests that the target blood pressure is <140/80 mmHg for all patients, irrespective of age. However, this statement

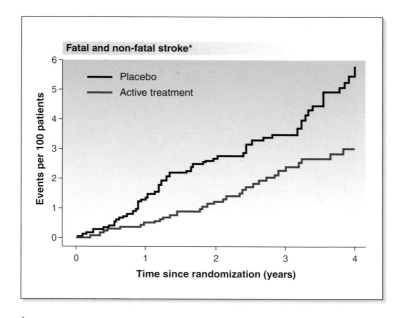

Fatal and non-fatal stroke*

▲

Fig. 11.3 Effect of treatment in subjects with isolated systolic hypertension. Results of the SystEur Study of a long-acting calcium-channel blocker in older subjects with isolated systolic hypertension. *$P = 0.003$. (From Staessen *et al* 1997, with permission of Elsevier Science.)

fails to recognize that isolated systolic hypertension, which is predominantly detected in the elderly, has a different pathophysiological basis from that of essential hypertension, which is largely a disease of younger people. Moreover, most physicians can testify to the difficulty of treating isolated systolic hypertension. Furthermore, data from three placebo-controlled trials indicate that a fall of just 10/5 mmHg is sufficient to reduce the risk of a cardiovascular event by a third. Therefore, relatively modest reductions in blood pressure are certainly worthwhile and it may be more appropriate in clinical practice to aim for 140/80 in patients who start out at ≤160 mmHg, but aim for a ≥20 mmHg reduction if the initial blood pressure is higher.

11.11 Are there dangers in reducing blood pressure?

 Some adverse effects, including postural hypotension and dizziness, can occur with the majority of antihypertensive medication, whilst others are drug-specific, e.g. bronchospasm with β-blockers and gout with thiazide. However, the available evidence would suggest that adverse events are no more common in the elderly than in younger hypertensive subjects.

Moreover, several trials have failed to find any difference in symptom scores or quality of life measures between subjects randomized to active therapy and those taking placebo (O'Donnell *et al* 1997). It is noteworthy that non-cardiovascular mortality is not significantly increased by therapy. Thus the concerns expressed by many physicians that any benefit from antihypertensive medication in the elderly will be offset by an excess of side-effects, such as falls, seem largely unjustified. However, it may be appropriate to start with lower doses in the elderly and then to titrate against response and symptoms.

11.12 Which drugs are effective?

A wealth of evidence supports the view that thiazide diuretics should be first-line therapy for hypertension in the elderly (*Fig. 7.3*). Thiazides are, in general, well tolerated and effective when given at low doses (e.g. bendroflumethiazide (bendrofluazide) 2.5 mg per day), and are inexpensive. However, they are ineffective if there is renal impairment or concomitant use of non-steroidal anti-inflammatory drugs (*see Q. 7.13*). In such circumstances long-acting dihydropyridine calcium-channel blockers may be a suitable alternative. However, short-acting drugs should not be used.

The STOP-2 trial compared newer (angiotensin-converting enzyme inhibitors and calcium-channel blockers) with older drugs (thiazides and β-blockers) in elderly antihypertensives and found no real difference between agents (*Table 11.2*) (Hansson *et al* 1999). However a meta-analysis implies that β-blockers may be less efficacious than thiazides in the elderly (*Table 11.3*) (Messerli *et al* 1998), which was also observed in the MRC trial in the elderly (*Fig. 7.3*). Potent vasodilators such as α-blockers and minoxidil should be used with care in older subjects with systolic hypertension as they may induce postural hypotension and lower diastolic pressure, thus impoverishing coronary artery perfusion, without having much impact on systolic blood pressure.

Trial data indicate that many patients (approximately two-thirds) will require combination therapy to reach target, and suitable combinations are discussed in Chapter 7 (*Q. 7.3*).

11.13 Is compliance with therapy a problem in the elderly?

In general, antihypertensive therapy is as well tolerated in the elderly as it is in younger patients (*see Q. 11.11*). Indeed, withdrawal rates from placebo-controlled clinical trials are comparable between placebo and active groups, and new and old drugs seem to be equally well tolerated. However, polypharmacy is an issue amongst older patients, and can reduce patient compliance. The use of combination therapy and rational prescribing habits can help minimize the number of drugs taken, as may the use of once-a-day formulations.

TABLE 11.2 Results of the STOP-2 study comparing thiazides and β-blockers (conventional) with calcium-channel blockers and ACE inhibitors (new); there was no difference in any of the outcome measures

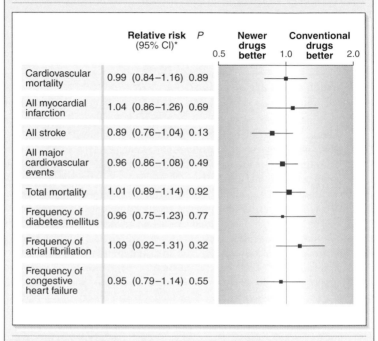

	Relative risk (95% CI)*	P
Cardiovascular mortality	0.99 (0.84–1.16)	0.89
All myocardial infarction	1.04 (0.86–1.26)	0.69
All stroke	0.89 (0.76–1.04)	0.13
All major cardiovascular events	0.96 (0.86–1.08)	0.49
Total mortality	1.01 (0.89–1.14)	0.92
Frequency of diabetes mellitus	0.96 (0.75–1.23)	0.77
Frequency of atrial fibrillation	1.09 (0.92–1.31)	0.32
Frequency of congestive heart failure	0.95 (0.79–1.14)	0.55

From Hansson *et al* 1999, with permission of Elsevier Science.

11.14 What about the very elderly?

There is less evidence concerning the benefits of blood pressure reduction in the over-80s. However, around 15% of patients included in six major trials in this area were aged over 80 years, and a recent meta-analysis concluded that antihypertensive treatment was effective in reducing cardiovascular morbidity, but not mortality, in subjects aged over 80 years (Gueyffier *et al* 1999). The HYVET study will directly address this increasingly important issue but until then it would seem appropriate to treat the very elderly who are otherwise well and have a reasonable quality of life.

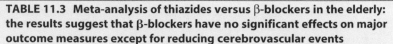

TABLE 11.3 Meta-analysis of thiazides versus β-blockers in the elderly: the results suggest that β-blockers have no significant effects on major outcome measures except for reducing cerebrovascular events

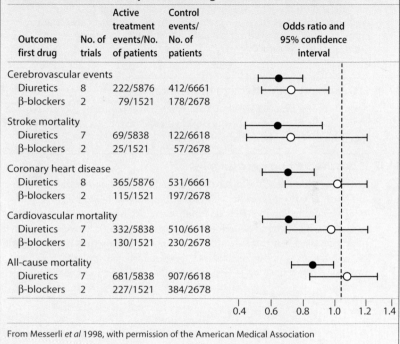

Outcome first drug	No. of trials	Active treatment events/No. of patients	Control events/ No. of patients	Odds ratio and 95% confidence interval
Cerebrovascular events				
Diuretics	8	222/5876	412/6661	
β-blockers	2	79/1521	178/2678	
Stroke mortality				
Diuretics	7	69/5838	122/6618	
β-blockers	2	25/1521	57/2678	
Coronary heart disease				
Diuretics	8	365/5876	531/6661	
β-blockers	2	115/1521	197/2678	
Cardiovascular mortality				
Diuretics	7	332/5838	510/6618	
β-blockers	2	130/1521	230/2678	
All-cause mortality				
Diuretics	7	681/5838	907/6618	
β-blockers	2	227/1521	384/2678	

0.4   0.6   0.8   1.0   1.2   1.4

From Messerli *et al* 1998, with permission of the American Medical Association

11.15 How common is postural hypotension?

> Postural hypotension may be defined as a fall in blood pressure, after 1–3 minutes of standing, of >20/10 mmHg. It is relatively common in the elderly, with estimates of ~5–20% in unselected populations, but much lower values reported amongst the 'healthy elderly'. Most antihypertensive drugs can induce, or worsen, postural hypotension but the problem seems much more common with vasodilators such as α-blockers and hydralazine. Angiotensin-converting enzyme inhibitors (ACEi) and calcium-channel blockers do not seem to induce postural hypotension, possibly because they preserve the normal reflex increase in peripheral vascular resistance on standing,

but they can worsen a pre-existing fall in blood pressure on standing. At low doses, postural hypotension is relatively uncommon with thiazides and β-blockers, but can occur. Nevertheless, in subjects with marked symptomatic postural hypotension who are receiving antihypertensive drugs it may be worthwhile withdrawing therapy and reassessing the situation before trying alternative agents or different drug combinations.

11.16 Is treatment cost-effective in the elderly?

Several studies have shown that antihypertensive treatment is cost-effective in the elderly, especially when relatively inexpensive drugs such as thiazides and β-blockers are used (Jackson 1998).

11.17 Is dose reduction necessary?

 With most agents such as β-blockers and angiotensin-converting enzyme inhibitors (ACEi) it is prudent to reduce the starting dose and then to titrate-up guided by the clinical response and occurrence of adverse events (e.g. start with 25 mg of atenolol and increase to 50 mg). However, with other agents such as thiazide diuretics no dose adjustment is necessary, but one should be aware that electrolyte abnormalities may be more pronounced and have more functional impact in older individuals.

Hypertension in women

12

THE ORAL CONTRACEPTIVE PILL (OCP)

12.1   Does the OCP cause hypertension?

 The OCP, by virtue of its oestrogen content, is a very important cause of secondary hypertension in women (Task Force on Oral Contraceptives 1999). A review of the data suggests that most women taking an OCP will experience a small, but detectable, increase in both systolic and diastolic blood pressures. Correspondingly, the prevalence of hypertension amongst users is two to three times that of age-matched women not taking the OCP; the risk of hypertension increases with age, duration of OCP use, baseline blood pressure, and body mass index. Early studies suggested that systolic and diastolic blood pressures rise by 5–6 mmHg and 1–2 mmHg respectively. The ethinylestradiol dose in current OCPs is lower (often 25–30 μg) than that used previously, and the rise in blood pressure and corresponding risk of hypertension may be lower. The available data suggest a strong relationship between oestrogen content and blood pressure, whereas the relationship between exogenous progestogen content and blood pressure rise is less clear.

12.2   What is the mechanism of OCP-related hypertension?

 The mechanisms that mediate raised blood pressure in response to OCP use are unclear. It is likely that several different factors are involved, including increased body mass, increased circulating fluid volume, peripheral insulin resistance, enhanced angiotensin II activity, and production of the vasoconstrictor endothelin-1. Animal models strongly support the role of renin–angiotensin–aldosterone system activation; oestrogen administration causes raised concentrations of angiotensinogen and angiotensin II, and the associated rise in blood pressure is attenuated by angiotensin-converting enzyme inhibitor treatment.

12.3   Does the incidence of OCP-related hypertension vary between preparations?

 The effects of OCP use on blood pressure are dependent on the oestrogen and progesterone content of the preparation. The OCP-induced rise in blood pressure correlates with oestrogen content so that the anticipated increase due to modern, low-dose OCPs (25–30 μg ethinylestradiol) is likely to be smaller. OCPs containing only progesterone, and parenteral progestogen treatments, do not appear to cause elevation of blood pressure, and may therefore be a suitable alternative means of contraception for those women in whom OCP-induced hypertension occurs (Bigrigg et al 1999). The overall incidence of OCP-induced hypertension is ~5% (Chasan-Taber et al 1996).

12.4 Can hypertensive women take the OCP?

Although it is advisable to avoid using the OCP in women with pre-existing hypertension, this is not always practical. Other means of contraception should be explored, and this modality should only be considered for carefully selected patients in whom the potential risks of pregnancy outweigh the risks of mild hypertension. Only low-dose OCP preparations should be used, if possible, and blood pressure response to treatment should be closely monitored.

12.5 How often should women on the OCP have their blood pressure checked?

Generally, blood pressure should be checked at 6-monthly intervals for the duration of treatment; this is facilitated by dispensing no more than 6 months' supply of OCP without a medical appointment. Screening should be maintained indefinitely because the risk of hypertension is linked to the duration of treatment, with greatest apparent risk after 6 or more years (Chasan-Taber 1996).

12.6 When should the OCP be stopped?

If blood pressure rises, then a decision to discontinue OCP treatment should be based on the degree of hypertension, overall cardiovascular risk profile, and potential risks of pregnancy. In general, treatment should be discontinued if systolic and/or diastolic blood pressure rises above 160 and 100 mmHg, respectively.

12.7 Does blood pressure return to normal after stopping the OCP?

In many cases, withdrawal of OCP treatment will lead to gradual blood pressure reduction over a period of 2–6 weeks. Blood pressure may fail to normalize after discontinuation, which may be due to the underlying progressive rise in blood pressure associated with advancing age, depending on the duration of treatment.

About 3% of women taking the OCP may develop reversible hypertension due to sensitivity to angiotensin, and these women are also at risk of developing pregnancy-induced hypertension.

12.8 What if the blood pressure does not normalize after withdrawing the OCP?

In some cases, hypertension persists after withdrawal of the OCP, even if there appears to be a close temporal relationship between commencing OCP and subsequent rise in blood pressure. Although a small number of patients will experience some reduction in blood pressure over a prolonged period, the majority are likely to have underlying essential hypertension. It is prudent to avoid reintroducing OCP treatment, so alternative means of contraception should be considered. Blood pressure should be managed in the same manner as de novo hypertension, and the association with prior OCP use should not detract from the importance of investigating for another possible underlying cause of hypertension, where appropriate (*see Ch. 9*).

PREGNANCY

12.9 What happens to blood pressure in a normal pregnancy?

There are a number of important haemodynamic changes that occur in pregnancy, which are thought to be mediated by increased circulating sex hormone concentrations, and partly due to the effects of the placenta on regional blood flow. Overall, there is a reduction in peripheral vascular resistance and an accompanying fall in blood pressure, which is greatest during the second trimester. Indeed, circulating fluid volume, cardiac output, renal blood flow and glomerular filtration rate are also increased. Enhanced vascular production of nitric oxide and prostacyclin have been found, which could account for the fall in systemic vascular resistance and improved renal blood flow.

12.10 How is hypertension in pregnancy defined?

Hypertension in pregnancy is defined as either an absolute blood pressure of greater than 140 mmHg systolic and/or 90 mmHg diastolic, or an increase of 25 mmHg and/or 15 mmHg respectively from pre-conception or first trimester blood pressures.

12.11 What is the incidence of hypertension in pregnancy?

Hypertension affects 5–10% of all pregnancies. It is second only to thromboembolic disease as a leading cause of maternal death, and poses a significant morbidity and mortality risk to the fetus.

12.12 What forms of hypertension occur in pregnancy?

There are several important forms of hypertension that occur in pregnancy, as outlined in Table 12.1.

12.13 What are the risks of hypertension in pregnancy?

The risks of hypertension can be considered as those which affect the mother or the developing fetus. Maternal risks are predominantly manifest in the cerebrovascular, cardiac and renal circulations and include significant increases in the occurrence of stroke (ischaemic and haemorrhagic), cardiac arrhythmia, ischaemic heart disease, and progressive and acute renal failure. Risks to the fetus are predominantly due to impaired uteroplacental blood flow, and include premature delivery, growth retardation, and death.

TABLE 12.1 Types of hypertension in pregnancy (Feldman 2001)

Type	Description
Chronic hypertension	≥140/90 mmHg prior to pregnancy or 20th week of gestation Also used to describe hypertension diagnosed during pregnancy that does not resolve postpartum
Pre-eclampsia	Multisystem disorder, including proteinuria, vasospasm and coagulation abnormalities
Pre-eclampsia superimposed on chronic hypertension	
Gestational hypertension*	≥140/90 mmHg or ≥30/15 mmHg rise in absence of pre-eclampsia, where BP returns to normal postpartum

*Also called pregnancy-induced or pregnancy-associated hypertension.

12.14 What is pre-eclampsia?

Pre-eclampsia is a syndrome unique to pregnancy that is characterized by reduced organ perfusion because of vasospasm, and activation of the coagulation cascade. It is diagnosed when blood pressure after the 20th week gestation is greater than 140 mmHg systolic and/or 90 mmHg diastolic, or rises more than 30 mmHg and/or 15 mmHg respectively above first trimester blood pressures. It is usually accompanied by proteinuria of at least 0.3 g/day and oedema, which is typically non-dependent and often located in the hands and face. Clinical manifestations of severe pre-eclampsia are given in Box 12.1.

Patients with existing hypertension are at increased risk of developing pre-eclampsia, and there may be some difficulty distinguishing pre-eclampsia from worsening of existing chronic hypertension. Factors that suggest pre-eclampsia superimposed on chronic hypertension are given in Box 12.2.

BOX 12.1 Clinical features of severe pre-eclampsia

- Systolic blood pressure ≥160 mmHg
- Diastolic blood pressure ≥110 mmHg
- Elevated serum creatinine (ischaemic nephropathy)
- Elevated transaminases (hepatocellular dysfunction)
- Microangiopathic haemolysis
- Thrombocytopenia
- Pulmonary oedema
- Oliguria (<500 ml/day)
- Intrauterine growth restriction
- HELLP syndrome (haemolysis, elevated liver enzymes, low platelet count)
- Seizures (eclampsia)

BOX 12.2 Features of pre-eclampsia in chronic hypertension

Clinical features that may help distinguish development of pre-eclampsia rather than worsening of chronic hypertension:

- New-onset proteinuria where absent prior to 20 weeks' gestation
- Sudden increase in proteinuria
- Sudden worsening of blood pressure control
- New abnormal laboratory values (esp. low platelet count)

12.15 Is blood pressure always raised in pre-eclampsia?

Raised blood pressure and proteinuria are hallmark diagnostic features of pre-eclampsia. However, because of the complex aetiology of the disorder, attempts to define a cut-off blood pressure, across a continuously distributed range, will be somewhat arbitrary. A further difficult aspect of using blood pressure to define pre-eclampsia is in distinguishing between pathological and physiological changes in blood pressure that occur normally during pregnancy (see Q. 12.9). The characteristic fall in blood pressure that occurs in the second trimester may partly obscure hypertension if pre-eclampsia develops during this period.

Overall, pre-eclampsia can be defined on the basis of hypertension and proteinuria, in association with several other clinical manifestations. In a very small number of cases, pre-eclampsia can be diagnosed when proteinuria and clinical and laboratory manifestations are strongly indicative, despite blood pressure appearing normal.

12.16 How often should blood pressure be assessed in pregnancy?

Blood pressure should be recorded at the first antenatal visit, and at every subsequent antenatal visit, typically every 4 weeks until 28 or 30 weeks; every 2 weeks until 36 weeks; and weekly after that. If a high reading (≥140 mmHg systolic and/or ≥90 mmHg diastolic) is obtained, blood pressure should be rechecked in 4–6 hours, and urinalysis performed. If an isolated high blood pressure recording is found, patients should be advised to rest supine, and require close monitoring for at least 48 hours. If blood pressure remains elevated, and/or other features suggest the possibility of pre-eclampsia, e.g. proteinuria, then patients should be considered for referral to the local obstetric unit for close observation and control of blood pressure.

12.17 Does hypertension in pregnancy run in families?

Hypertension in pregnancy, including pre-eclampsia, does appear to run in families in certain cases; the risks are higher in those patients with a positive family history in a first-degree relative (Roberts & Cooper 2001). However, genetic analysis is difficult to study, because the condition inherently only affects women who have reproduced. In pre-eclampsia there is a lack of concordance between monozygotic twins, and increased risk due to change of paternity, both suggesting fetal, rather than maternal, factors may be important. Some groups support the hypothesis that a single gene with incomplete penetrance, or whose expression is pregnancy-specific, could be acting in the mother (*see also Q. 9.61*). Overall, the risk of developing pre-eclampsia appears more closely related to other factors (*Q. 12.22*) than family history.

12.18 What is the risk of hypertension in a subsequent pregnancy?

Pre-eclampsia is more likely to happen in a second pregnancy if a woman has suffered it before. Mild pre-eclampsia at term is less likely to recur (5–10%) and when it does it is usually mild again. After severe pre-eclampsia, the recurrence rate is about 20–25% in subsequent pregnancies. After eclampsia, about 25–30% of subsequent pregnancies will be complicated by pre-eclampsia, but only 2% with eclampsia again.

12.19 How long does blood pressure take to return to normal after delivery?

Blood pressure would be expected to return to normal soon after delivery, usually within the first 2 weeks. In severe pre-eclampsia, or eclampsia, delivery is often the treatment of choice.

12.20 Is there a greater risk of hypertension in later life?

Chronic hypertension is more common after pre-eclampsia, affecting about

15% at 2 years. It is even more likely after eclampsia or severe pre-eclampsia (especially if recurrent or occurring during the second trimester), affecting 30–50% of women.

12.21 What is the mechanism of hypertension in pregnancy?

The precise mechanisms remain unclear. In gestational hypertension, the rise in blood pressure may be an exaggerated physiological response to the enlarged circulating fluid volume, characterized by increased cardiac output and widened pulse pressure. In pre-eclampsia there is evidence of widespread vascular dysfunction, such that production of nitric oxide and prostacyclin is significantly impaired, and thromboxane A_2 production increases unchecked (Bernheim 1997). The latter predisposes to vascular occlusion and tissue ischaemia, while the former contributes to vasospasm, reduced blood flow and increased systemic blood pressure.

12.22 Who is at increased risk?

Several factors are known to be associated with increased risk of developing pre-eclampsia (*Box 12.3*).

12.23 What are the aims of treatment?

The aims of treatment are to lower blood pressure as safely and as effectively as possible, thereby reducing the potential risks to mother and fetus (Brown & Whitworth 1999). Where hypertension is severe, typically with systolic blood pressure of 170 mmHg or more, there is general agreement that blood pressure should be reduced as a matter of urgency to protect against the risks of maternal stroke and eclampsia. Blood pressure

---

BOX 12.3 Risk factors for pre-eclampsia

- First pregnancy
- Pre-eclampsia in a previous pregnancy
- Age under 20 years or over 35 years
- Short stature
- Change of partner
- Migraine
- Family history of pre-eclampsia or eclampsia
- Previous hypertension
- Raynaud's disease
- Underweight
- Systemic lupus erythematosus (SLE)
- Multiple pregnancy (e.g. twins)
- Hydatidiform mole

reduction is one of the most important aspects of pre-eclampsia management; however, delivery is the definitive treatment.

12.24 What is the target blood pressure?

The target systolic and diastolic blood pressures are 140 and 90 mmHg respectively. Some advocate lower target pressures; however, there is little clinical evidence to support this.

12.25 Which drugs are contraindicated in pregnancy?

 The vast majority of antihypertensive drugs available in the UK do not have a license for use in pregnancy, and prescribers should be particularly aware of their responsibility to ensure that the risks of drug administration in pregnancy are justifiably offset by risk reduction attained by blood pressure control.

ACE inhibitors are known to cause oligohydramnios, impaired fetal renal function and neonatal anuria, and are therefore contraindicated in pregnancy. β-blockers can cause intrauterine growth retardation when used in early pregnancy, but their use appears to be safe during the third trimester. A recent Cochrane Collaboration Systematic Review found that diazoxide is associated with profound hypotension, and should, therefore, be avoided.

12.26 Which drugs can be used?

 Drugs that have accumulated efficacy and safety data in pregnancy include methyldopa and hydralazine (Dekker & Sibai 2001). However, the latter is now rarely used in a non-emergency setting. The β-blocker labetolol is licensed for use in pregnancy and is usually well tolerated. Other β-blockers are sometimes used but may be best avoided in earlier stages of pregnancy because of the risk of fetal growth retardation. Calcium-channel blockers, particularly nifedipine, are effective in rapidly controlling high blood pressure and appear to be well tolerated; however, their safety profile with regard to the developing fetus has not yet been adequately evaluated. As outlined above (Q. 12.25), ACE inhibitors should be avoided owing to excess fetal risk, and it is prudent to avoid angiotensin II receptor antagonists unless clear evidence of efficacy and safety become available.

12.27 What is the role of aspirin?

Research in the past has identified some major risk factors for pre-eclampsia, and manipulation of these, including prostaglandins, might result in a decrease in its frequency. In the early 1990s aspirin was thought to offer particular benefits in secondary prevention of pre-eclampsia; however, large trials have shown that this is not the case (Livingston & Sibai 2001). The only patients in whom any benefit was derived were those at a very high risk of developing severe early-onset disease. Prophylactic low-dose aspirin started early in pregnancy in women with chronic hypertension is not effective in reducing the frequency of superimposed pre-eclampsia and should be avoided (Dekker & Sibai 2001).

12.28 Who should be referred for specialist management?

Patients with hypertension in pregnancy should be referred for specialist management if there is poor blood pressure control, new onset of proteinuria or other features suggesting pre-eclampsia, or there is suspicion of intrauterine growth retardation.

HORMONE REPLACEMENT THERAPY (HRT)

12.29 Does HRT cause increased blood pressure?

 A recent randomized, placebo-controlled study of oestrogen and combined oestrogen–progesterone HRT preparations found that there was no apparent effect of HRT treatment on systolic blood pressure. Furthermore, oestrogen was associated with beneficial cardiovascular effects on lipid and coagulation profiles. HRT does not appear to cause a general increase in systemic blood pressure (Writing Group for the PEPI Trial 1995). However, idiosyncratic rises in blood pressure have been reported in several cases; therefore it is prudent to monitor blood pressure response to treatment two to three times within the first 6 months, and at least every 6 months thereafter.

12.30 Should HRT be withheld in women with hypertension?

There is no absolute contraindication to HRT in women with established hypertension, and the risks of treatment should be considered, for each patient, in the context of potential benefits. Ideally, blood pressure should be controlled before initiating HRT, and carefully monitored thereafter. If there is a significant rise in blood pressure, or control worsens, HRT should be temporarily discontinued to assess its contribution. Clearly, the decision to administer HRT will be heavily influenced by the desire to control postmenopausal symptoms, osteoporosis risk, patient choice and perceptions of health benefits. The absolute cardiovascular benefit achieved by HRT appears to be substantially offset by increased thromboembolic disease risk in unselected patients (Hulley *et al* 1998), although there may be greater potential benefits in hypertensive patients, who have higher cardiovascular risk.

PATIENT QUESTIONS

12.31 Can I become pregnant if I have high blood pressure?

In almost all cases the answer is yes, as long as you first consult your doctor. It may be necessary to change your medication, as you should not become pregnant on certain tablets, and your doctor may also suggest referral to a hypertension specialist. Sometime, it is advisable to first control high blood pressure before becoming pregnant.

12.32 What is the chance of getting hypertension on the Pill?

Overall the risks of developing hypertension due to the contraceptive pill are about 1 in 20. However, some of these women would have developed hypertension anyway. Therefore, it is important to ensure that you have your blood pressure checked every 6 months whilst taking the pill.

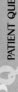

Other issues

13

RACIAL ISSUES

13.1 Do Afro-Caribbeans have an increased risk of the complications of hypertension?

Although hypertension is extremely prevalent world-wide, the number of hypertensive Afro-Caribbeans is disproportionately higher than their representation in the population as a whole. Hypertension in Afro-Caribbeans tends to appear earlier than in whites and is often not treated aggressively enough. The result is a higher prevalence of more severe hypertension in this ethnic group. Not only do Afro-Caribbeans have an increased risk of complications, but also when such complications recur they are more severe. This is true for cardiac involvement, and analysis of matched groups of black and white hypertensives have shown that blacks demonstrate an excessive rise in left ventricular mass index. Interestingly, the echocardiogram often shows patterns of increased left ventricular mass before the development of significant hypertension. Stroke is also an extremely common complication of hypertension in Afro-Caribbeans. It is estimated that death from stroke in this ethnic group is 66% higher than in whites. Renal disease is also more common and the risk of end-stage renal disease in one study was 4.2 times greater in blacks than in whites and the prevalence of hypertensive renal disease 17.7 times higher in Afro-Caribbeans than in whites.

13.2 Why are diuretics more effective than ACE inhibitors in Afro-Caribbeans?

Diuretics are more effective in Afro-Caribbeans, as this group tends to have low-renin, volume-expanded hypertension. Thus ACE inhibitors are less effective. The same is true for β-blockers, as these drugs also act, in part, via the renin–angiotensin system by decreasing renin release from the kidney. Interestingly, it is known that blacks have altered sodium handling compared to whites, and recently polymorphisms of the α-adducing gene have been associated with low-renin hypertension and altered sodium homeostasis. However, the question as to whether polymorphisms of this gene will explain why black Africans have low-renin hypertension remains unanswered.

13.3 Is malignant hypertension more common in certain ethnic groups?

There is no doubt that malignant hypertension is more common in black Africans. There are a number of possible reasons for this including racial differences in renal physiology and socioeconomic status. In addition, there are also differences in genetic and environmental characteristics. End-stage renal disease is also more common in black Africans and this condition is associated with malignant hypertension. Interestingly, although black Africans are especially prone to cerebral haemorrhage, they are less susceptible to the development of coronary artery disease; the reasons for this remain unclear.

13.4 Are there differences in response to therapy between racial groups?

Since black Africans tend towards low-renin volume-expanded hypertension, they respond very well to treatment with diuretics and also calcium-channel blockers. For the same reason they respond less well to ACE inhibition and β-blockade. In addition, racial differences in the β_2-adrenoceptor gene polymorphism may also influence response to β-blocker therapy in black populations.

CHILDREN

13.5 How should blood pressure be measured in children?

Blood pressure should be measured using a mercury or aneroid sphygmomanometer and appropriately sized cuff placed over the upper arm, where the bladder encircles 80–100% of the arm circumference and the width should be 40% of the upper arm circumference. An automated sphygmomanometer, such as the Dynamap device, can be used in infants and children who will not cooperate with manual measurements. It is suggested that children should be seated quietly for 5 minutes before obtaining measurements.

> Height is the most important factor accounting for blood pressure variability across childhood populations, in addition to age and weight, and therefore blood pressure is most appropriately expressed as a centile for any given patient height (*Fig. 13.1*). Normal blood pressure is defined as <90th centile, 'high-normal' between the 90th and 95th centiles, and abnormal blood pressure at the 95th centile or beyond. To establish the diagnosis of hypertension, at least three abnormal readings should be obtained on separate occasions.

13.6 How common is hypertension in children?

Hypertension in children is comparatively rare, and more likely to be associated with an underlying medical disorder, especially when blood pressure is very high. It is very rarely diagnosed in children less than 5 years of age, with the frequency increasing beyond 10 years of age (Lauer & Clarke 1989, Temple & Nahata 2000). A recent Medline review of

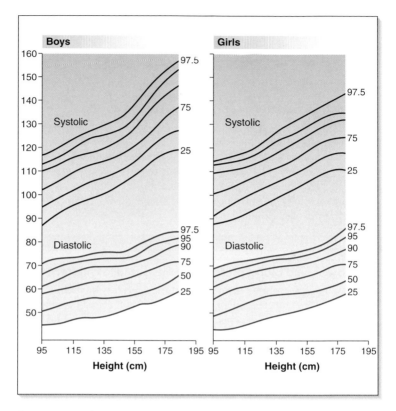

▲

Fig. 13.1 Systolic and diastolic blood pressure by centile, in boys and girls, by subject height. (From de Swiet M *et al* 1989, with permission of the BMJ Publishing Group.)

randomized and non-randomized paediatric studies indicates that the overall incidence of hypertension in the child population is 1–3%.

Some children show a pattern of intermittently elevated blood pressure (beyond the 95th centile) and, in general, they are otherwise healthy with no underlying renal, cardiac or other organ disease. There is no clear consensus on the appropriateness of follow-up for children with this pattern of blood pressure, although longitudinal studies have identified a fourfold increase in the risk of adult hypertension in this group.

13.7 What is the incidence of secondary hypertension in children?

Unlike adult hypertension, most cases in childhood are secondary to some underlying medical disorder. Essential hypertension becomes increasingly

TABLE 13.1 Causes of childhood hypertension by age group

	Infants	School-age	Adolescents
Primary/essential	<1%	15–30%	85–95%
Secondary	99%	70–85%	5–15%
Renal parenchymal disease	20%	60–70%	
Renovascular	25%	5–10%	
Endocrine	1%	3–5%	
Aortic coarctation	35%	10–20%	
Reflux nephropathy	0%	5–10%	
Neoplastic	4%	1–5%	
Miscellaneous	20%	1–5%	

From Flynn 2001, with permission of Elsevier Science.

prevalent with advancing age, such that it is the most common form among older adolescents (*Table 13.1*).

13.8 When should children be screened for hypertension?

Although hypertension in childhood is rare, the high likelihood of identifying an underlying medical cause justifies some degree of blood pressure screening. Sick children should have their blood pressure measured whenever a general medical examination is indicated. In addition, certain high-risk groups should have regular blood pressure measurements (*Box 13.1*). At present, however, general population screening for childhood hypertension is not recommended.

13.9 What drugs can be used safely in children?

As in adults, management should incorporate non-pharmacological measures such as weight loss, aerobic exercise, and dietary modification including sodium restriction. Despite several studies that have reported efficacy and safety data in children, there is a lack of evidence from randomized clinical trials to guide the choice of antihypertensive agent. Further caveats arise in that paediatric dosing regimens are often

BOX 13.1 Indications for blood pressure measurement in childhood (de Swiet *et al* 1989)

- Opportunistically in unwell children
- Where a high reading has been noted previously
- History of kidney, bladder or ureter disease
- Those with diabetes
- Family history of hypertension (less compelling)

unavailable and, of those that are available, most relate to older antihypertensive drugs that have fallen out of favour in adult hypertension. In general, calcium-channel blockers, angiotensin-converting enzyme inhibitors, diuretics and β-blockers appear safe and effective. Specific drug characteristics will determine the suitability for individual patients; for example, diuretics may be unsatisfactory in a teenage athlete. In the setting of emergency antihypertensive treatment, intravenous labetolol, sodium nitroprusside and nicardipine are all effective. Liaison with the local pharmacy department will be important in ensuring that drugs can be supplied in dosages determined by patient weight, and prepared in elixir form in certain cases.

13.10　What is pseudohypertension of youth?

Pseudohypertension is used to describe the characteristic pattern of systolic hypertension in young people (<30 years), who have normal aortic blood pressure (O'Rourke *et al* 2000). This results from an exaggeration of the normal amplification of blood pressure from the aorta to the arm, owing to an unknown mechanism, but possibly related to unusually distensible arteries. Subjects are usually young, tall fit men. Often brachial diastolic and mean arterial pressures are normal. Patients with pseudohypertension have not been subject to long-term follow-up, but it is not thought to be associated with any increased risk of hypertension or cardiovascular risk. Nevertheless, subjects suspected of pseudohypertension should be referred to a specialist centre for further investigation and/or confirmation of the diagnosis.

FUTURE DEVELOPMENTS

13.11　What new drugs are likely to emerge for the treatment of hypertension?

Hypertension is a common disorder, and a number of drug companies have an active drug discovery programme in this area. The likely new classes of compound which will appear in the near future include vasopeptidase inhibitors (which inhibit both angiotensin-inverting enzyme and neutral endopeptidase), endothelin-antagonists, and combined angiotensin-inverting and endothelin-converting enzyme inhibitors. Whether these drugs will reach market depends on a number of factors, not least safety and tolerability, but some of them have shown promise in early clinical trials, as useful new agents. Obviously as new peptides and regulatory systems are discovered, then it is likely that new agonists and antagonists to these will be developed in order to modulate blood pressure. Finally, isolated systolic hypertension is at present treated with drugs which are really developed for essential hypertension. Therefore, it provides an interesting opportunity for new drugs to be developed specifically to target the pathogenesis of this condition—namely large artery stiffening. Although nitrates have potential use in this area, overcoming tolerance and developing other novel therapies, it is likely to occupy many pharmaceutical companies for some time.

Appendix: Useful addresses and web sites

General

British Hypertension Society
Blood Pressure Unit
Department of Medicine
St George's Medical School
London SW17 0RE
Tel: 020 8725 3412
Fax: 020 8725 2959
Email: bhsis@sghms.ac.uk
http://www.hyp.ac.uk/bhs/

International Society for Hypertension in Blacks (US)
2045 Manchester Street
NE
Atlanta
Georgia 30324
http://www.ishib.org/main/ishib_open.htm

European Society of Hypertension
http://www.eshonline.org/

World Hypertension League
http://www.mco.edu/org/whl/index.html

Primary Care Cardiovascular Society
36 Berrymede Road
London W4 5JD
Tel: 020 8994 8775
Fax: 020 8742 2130
http://www.pccs.org.uk/

British Association for Nursing in Cardiac Care (BANCC)
c/o British Cardiac Society
9 Fitzroy Square
London W1T 5HW
Tel: 020 7692 5413/020 7383 3887
Fax: 020 7383 5961

Charities, patient organisations and support groups
Blood Pressure Association
60 Cranmer Terrace

London SW17 0QS
Tel: 020 8772 4994
Fax : 020 8772 4999
http://www.bpassoc.org.uk/

British Cardiac Patients Association
100 Anerley Road
London SE19 2AN
Tel: 020 8289 5591
Fax: 020 8289 5592
Email: bcpa@easynet.co.uk
http://www.cardiac-bcpa.co.uk

British Heart Foundation
14 Fitzhardinge Street
London W1H 6DH
Tel: 020 7935 0185
Fax: 020 7486 5820
Email: internet@bhf.org.uk
http://www.bhf.org.uk/

BHF Centre of Physical Activity and Health
http://www.bhfactive.org.uk

American Heart Association
National Center
7272 Greenville Avenue
Dallas
TX 75231
http://www.americanheart.org/

Irish Heart Foundation
Head Office Address:
4 Clyde Road
Ballsbridge
Dublin 4
Tel: 01 6685001
Fax: 01 6685896
Email: info@irishheart.ie
http://www.irishheart.ie/happyheart/

Heartlink (UK & Overseas Heart Society)
25 Close Street
Hemsworth
Pontefract
West Yorkshire WF9 4QP
Tel: 01977 625656

UK Freephone: 0500 676 670
Email: support@heartlink.org.uk
http://www.heartlink.org.uk/

Chest, Heart & Stroke Scotland
65 North Castle Street
Edinburgh EH2 3LT
Tel: 0131 225 6963
Fax: 0131 220 6313
Helpline: 0845 077 6000
Contact Name: Jo Bennett, Director of Health Promotion
Email: admin@chss.org.uk
http://www.chss.org.uk/

Northern Ireland Chest, Heart & Stroke Association
21 Dublin Road
Belfast BT2 7HB
Tel: 028 9032 0184
Fax: 028 9033 3487
Advice Helpline: 084 5769 7299
Cardiac Liaison Sister Helpline: 084 5601 1658
http://www.nichsa.com/

The Stroke Association
Stroke House
123 Whitecross Street
London EC1Y 8JJ
Tel: 020 7566 0300
Fax: 020 7490 2686
Helpline: 0845 30 33 100
Email: informationservice@stroke.org.uk
http://www.stroke.org.uk/

Heart and Stroke Foundation of Canada
http://ww1.heartandstroke.ca/

Action Heart
Wellesley House
117 Wellington Road
Dudley DY1 1UB
Tel: 01384 230222
Fax: 01384 254437
Contact Name: Jeff Moore

Family Heart Association
7 North Road
Maidenhead

Berkshire SL6 1PE
Tel: 01628 628638
Fax: 01628 628698
Email: ad@familyheart.org
http://www.familyheart.org/

Diabetes UK
10 Parkway
London NW1 7AA
Tel: 020 7424 1000
Fax: 020 7424 1001
Email: info@diabetes.org.uk
http://www.diabetes.org.uk/

Action on Pre-eclampsia (APEC)
84–88 Pinner Road
Harrow
Middlesex HA1 4HZ
Tel: 020 8863 3271
Fax: 020 8424 0653
Email: enquiries@apec.org.uk
Helpline: 020 8427 4217 (weekdays 10 a.m. – 1 p.m.)
http://www.apec.org.uk

NHS – Giving up smoking
http://www.givingupsmoking.co.uk/

QuitsmokingUK.com (patient group)
http://www.quitsmokinguk.com/

QuitNet (US site)
http://www.quitnet.org/

Mended Hearts, Inc
US patient organization
http://mendedhearts.org/

British Cardiac Society
9 Fitzroy Square
London W1T 5HW
Tel: 020 7383 3887
Fax: 020 7388 0903
http://www.bcs.com/

National Heart Forum
Tavistock House South
Tavistock Square

London WC1H 9LG
Tel: 020 7383 7638
Fax: 020 7387 2799
Email: webenquiry@heartforum.org.uk
http://www.heartforum.org.uk/nationalheartforum.html

CORDA (The Coronary Artery Disease Research Association)
PO Box 9353
121 Sydney Street
London SW3 6ZA
Tel: 020 7349 8686
Fax: 020 7349 9414
http://www.corda.org.uk

Coronary Prevention Group
2 Taviton Street
London WC1H 0BT
Tel: 020 7927 2125
Fax: 020 7927 2127
http://www.healthnet.org.uk

LOCAL GROUPS

Cardiff Hypertension Multiple Risk Factor Intervention Clinic
http://www.mrfc2000fsnet.co.uk

Doncaster Heart Support Group
http://www.geocities.com/donheartuk/index.html

Great Yarmouth & Waveney HeartCare Cardiac Support Group
http://www.heartcarecsg.co.uk

Heart Throbs HSG (North London, Middlesex and Hertfordshire areas)
http://www.heart-throbs.org.uk

Heart to Herts Cardiac Support Group
http://www.heart-to-herts.co.uk

Heartbeat (East Suffolk Cardiac Support Group)
Tel: Len Tate (Hon Vice-President): 01206 393292
http://www.heartbeat.eastsuffolk.btinternet.co.uk/

Heartbeat'95 (Merthyr Tydfil)
http://www.heartbeat95.org.uk/

Mid-Cheshire Heart Support Group
http://www.communigate.co.uk/chesh/midcheshireheartsupportgroup

Milton Keynes Community Cardiac Group
http://www.mkcardiacgroup.org/

Redditch Hale and Hearties
http://www.redditchhaleandhearties.org.uk/

Salisbury Heart Group
http://www.salisburyheartgroup.org.uk

SHARP (Scottish Heart and Arterial disease Risk Prevention)
Ninewells Hospital
Dundee DD1 9SY
Tel: 01382 660 111
http://www.dundee.ac.uk/sharp

Solihull Heart Support Group
http://www.solihullheartsupport.org.uk

Government sites and guidelines
WHO/ISH guidelines
Revised guidelines will be posted here
http://www5.who.int/cardiovascular-diseases

UK National Service Framework for Coronary Heart Disease (2000)
http://www.doh.gov.uk/nsf/coronarych4.htm

CMO site
Source of Chief Medical Officer's publications, including 'The Expert Patient'
http://www.doh.gov.uk/cmo/publications.htm

Health Development Agency
Publications, including patient information sheets on heart disease, in Gujerati, Bengali, Hindi and Punjabi
http://www.hda-online.org.uk/html/resources/publications_a-q.html

National Electronic Library for Health (pilot site)
http://www.nelh.nhs.uk/

Heart Diseases Virtual Branch Library (pilot site)
http://www.wish-uk.org/znelh/

NHS Direct Health Encyclopaedia
http://www.nhsdirect.nhs.uk/nhsdoheso/index.asp

National Heart, Lung & Blood Institute (US)
http://www.nhlbi.nih.gov/hbp/index.html

Research
National Heart Research Fund (UK)
Suite 12D

Joseph's Well
Leeds LS3 1AB
Tel: 0113 234 7474
Fax: 0113 297 6208
Email: mail@heartresearch.org.uk
http://www.heartresearch.org.uk/

Framingham Heart Study
Part of the National Heart, Blood and Lung Institute, USA, developed
Framingham Heart Study Prediction Score Sheets
http://rover.nhlbi.nih.gov/about/framingham/

National Kidney Research Fund (UK)
Kings Chambers
Priestgate
Peterborough PE1 1FG
Tel: 01733 704650
Helpline: 0845 300 1499
Email: enquiries@nkrf.org.uk
http://www.nkrf.org.uk

UK National Institute of Health
Biomedical research, free
http://www.nih.gov/health

UK National Institute of Clinical Excellence
National Institute for Clinical Excellence
11 Strand
London WC2N 5HR
Tel: Main Reception: 020 7766 9191
Fax: Main Reception: 020 7766 9123
Email: nice@nice.nhs.uk
http://www.nice.org.uk

Patient information sites
Health in Focus
UK information site with GP-written patient information sheets on various
conditions, including hypertension, assessment of latest developments, and
useful links
http://www.healthinfocus.co.uk/

Net Doctor
UK patient information site
http://www.netdoctor.co.uk/diseases/facts/hypertension.htm

Medicine Net
US web site with patient information on common conditions, including high blood pressure
http://www.focusonhighbloodpressure.com/

Heart Information Network
US information web site for patients
Heartinfo.org
c/o Trigenesis Communications
26 Main Street
Chatham
NJ 07928
http://www.heartinfo.com/

Praxis
US patient and practitioner information
http://www.praxis.md

Surgery door
UK patient information
http://www.surgerydoor.co.uk/index.asp

Blood Pressure.com
http://www.bloodpressure.com/

British Nutrition Foundation
http://www.nutrition.org.uk/

American Dietetic Association
http://www.eatright.org/

US Food and Nutrition Information Center
http://www.nal.usda.gov/fnic/

My BP
http://www.mybp.com/

Journals

British Medical Journal (collection of articles on hypertension)
http://bmj.com/cgi/collection/hypertension

American Journal of Hypertension
http://www.medicinedirect.com/

Blood Pressure Monitoring
http://www.bpmonitoring.com/

Hypertension
http://hyper.ahajournals.org/

European Heart Journal
http://www.medicinedirect.com/

ACC Current Journal Review
http://www.cardiosource.com/

American Heart Journal
http://intl.elsevierhealth.com/journals/

American Journal of Cardiology
http://www.medicinedirect.com/

Cardiology in Review
http://www.cardiologyinreview.com/

Cardiovascular Research
http://www.medicinedirect.com/

Core Journals in Cardiology
http://www.elsevier.com/

International Journal of Cardiology
http://www.medicinedirect.com/

Journal of Cardiovascular Risk
http://www.jcardiovascularrisk.com/

Journal of Hypertension
http://www.jhypertension.com/

Stroke
http://stroke.ahajournals.org/

REFERENCES

Chapter 1

Bidlingmeyer I, Burnier M, Bidlingmeyer M 1996 Isolated office hypertension: a prehypertensive state? Journal of Hypertension 14: 327–332

Casiglia E, Palatini P 1998 Cardiovascular risk factors in the elderly. Journal of Human Hypertension 12: 575–581

Joint National Committee on Prevention, Detection, Evaluation and Treatment of High Blood Pressure 1997 The sixth report of the Joint National Committee on Prevention, Detection, Evaluation and Treatment of High Blood Pressure (JNC VI). Archives of Internal Medicine 157: 2413–2446

Khattar RS, Swales JD, Dore C et al 2001 Effect of aging on the prognostic significance of ambulatory systolic, diastolic, and pulse pressure in essential hypertension. Circulation 104: 783–789

Law CM, de Swiet M, Osmond C 1993 Initiation of hypertension in utero and its amplification throughout life. British Medical Journal 306: 24–27

McMahon S, Peto R, Cutler J et al 1990 Blood pressure, stroke, and coronary heart disease. Part 1, prolonged differences in blood pressure: prospective observational studies corrected for the regression dilution bias. Lancet 335: 765–774

Port S, Demer L, Jennrich R et al 2000 Systolic blood pressure and mortality. Lancet 355: 175–180

Rodgers A, Lawes C, MacMahon S 2000 Reducing the global burden of blood pressure-related cardiovascular disease. Journal of Hypertension 18: S3–S6

Rudd AG, Wolfe CD, Howard RS 1997 Prevention of neurological disease in later life. Journal of Neurology, Neurosurgery and Psychiatry 63(Suppl 1): S39–S52

Sagie A, Larson MG, Levy D 1993 The natural history of borderline isolated systolic hypertension. New England Journal of Medicine 329: 1912–1917

Strandberg TE, Salomaa V 2000 White coat effect, blood pressure and mortality in men: prospective cohort study. European Heart Journal 21: 1714–1718

Chapter 2

Bulpitt CJ, Palmer AJ, Fletcher AE et al 1995 Proportion of patients with isolated systolic hypertension who have burned-out diastolic hypertension. Journal of Human Hypertension 9: 675–678

Franklin SS, Gustin IVW, Wong ND et al 1997 Hemodynamic patterns of age-related changes in blood pressure: The Framingham Heart Study. Circulation 96: 308–315

Hypertension Prevention Trial Research Group 1990 The hypertension prevention trial. Three-year effects of dietary changes on blood pressure. Archives of Internal Medicine 150: 153–162

Marmot MG, Elliott P, Shipley MJ 1994 Alcohol and blood pressure: the INTERSALT study. British Medical Journal 308: 1263–1267

Mulrow CD, Chiquette E, Angel L et al 2000 Dieting to reduce body weight for controlling hypertension in adults. Cochrane Database of Systematic Reviews: CD000484

Rose G, Stamler J 1989 The INTERSALT study: background, methods and main results. INTERSALT Co-operative Research Group. Journal of Human Hypertension 3: 283–288

Staessen J, Amery A, Fagard R 1990 Isolated systolic hypertension in the elderly. Journal of Hypertension 8: 393–405

Stamler R, Stamler J, Riedlinger WF et al 1978 Weight and blood pressure. Findings in hypertension screening of 1 million Americans. Journal of the American Medical Association 240: 1607–1610

Thun MJ, Peto R, Lopez AD 1997 Alcohol consumption and mortality among middle-aged and elderly U.S. adults. New England Journal of Medicine 337: 1705–1714

Chapter 3

Dodson PM, Lip GY, Eames SM et al 1996 Hypertensive retinopathy: a review of existing classification systems and a suggestion for a simplified grading system. Journal of Human Hypertension 10: 93–98

Fang JJ, Alderman MH 2000 Serum uric acid and cardiovascular mortality the NHANES I epidemiological follow-up study, 1971–1992. National Health and Nutrition Examination Survey. Journal of the American Medical Association 283: 2404–2410

Hall IR, Tyrrell S, Wilkinson IB et al 2001 Self-referral multiple cardiovascular risk factor assessment – the Cardiff experience. British Journal of Cardiology 8: 303–310

Katz SM, Lavin L, Swartz C 1979 Glomerular lesions in benign essential hypertension. A study of eight biopsy specimens with laboratory evidence suggestive of glomerular abnormalities. Archives of Pathology & Laboratory Medicine 103: 199–203

Lip GY, Beevers M, Beevers DG 1995 Complications and survival of 315 patients with malignant-phase hypertension. Journal of Hypertension 13: 915–924

Waring WS, Webb DJ, Maxwell SR 2000 Uric acid as a risk factor for cardiovascular disease. Quarterly Journal of Medicine 93: 707–713

Weinstock BW, Keane WF 2001 Proteinuria and cardiovascular disease. American Journal of Kidney Diseases 38: S8–S13

Chapter 4

British Cardiac Society, British Hyperlipidaemia Association, British Hypertension Society, endorsed by the British Diabetic Association 1998 Joint British recommendations on prevention of coronary heart disease in clinical practice. Heart 80(Suppl 2): S1–29

Ramsay L, Williams B, Johnston G et al 1999 Guidelines for management of hypertension: report of the third working party of the British Hypertension Society. Journal of Human Hypertension 13: 569–592

Chapter 5

Greenland P, Smith JS Jr, Grundy SM 2001 Improving coronary heart disease risk assessment in asymptomatic people: role of traditional risk factors and noninvasive cardiovascular tests. Circulation 104: 1863–1867

Grundy SM, Pasternak R, Greenland P 1999 Assessment of cardiovascular risk by use of multiple-risk-factor assessment equations: a statement for healthcare professionals from the American Heart Association and the American College of Cardiology. Circulation 100: 1481–1492

Haffner S, Lehto S, Ronnemaa T 1998 Mortality from coronary heart disease in subjects with type 2 diabetes and in non-diabetic subjects with and without prior myocardial infarction. New England Journal of Medicine 339: 229–234

Ramsay LE, Williams B, Johnston GD 1999 Guidelines for management of hypertension: Report of the Third Working Party of the British Hypertension Society. Journal of Human Hypertension 13: 569–592

Chapter 6

Blumenthal JA, Sherwood A, Gullette EC et

al 2000 Exercise and weight loss reduce blood pressure in men and women with mild hypertension: effects on cardiovascular, metabolic, and hemodynamic functioning. Archives of Internal Medicine 160: 1947–1958

Cassano PA, Segal MR, Vokonas PS et al 1990 Body fat distribution, blood pressure, and hypertension. A prospective cohort study of men in the normative aging study. Annals of Epidemiology 1: 33–48

Erwteman TM, Nagelkerke N, Lubsen J et al 1984 Beta blockade, diuretics, and salt restriction for the management of mild hypertension: a randomised double blind trial. British Medical Journal 289: 406–409

Grimm RH Jr, Neaton JD, Elmer PJ 1990 The influence of oral potassium chloride on blood pressure in hypertensive men on a low-sodium diet. New England Journal of Medicine 322: 569–574

Gronbaek M, Deis A, Sorensen TI et al 1995 Mortality associated with moderate intakes of wine, beer, or spirits. British Medical Journal 310: 1165–1169

Higashi Y, Sasaki S, Kurisu S et al 1999 Regular aerobic exercise augments endothelium-dependent vascular relaxation in normotensive as well as hypertensive subjects: role of endothelium-derived nitric oxide. Circulation 100: 1194–1202

Kauhanen J, Kaplan GA, Goldberg DE et al 1997 Beer bingeing and mortality: results from the Kuopio ischaemic heart disease risk factor study, a prospective population based study. British Medical Journal 315: 846–851

Khaw KT, Barrett-Connor E 1987 Dietary potassium and stroke-associated mortality. A 12-year prospective population study. New England Journal of Medicine 316: 235–240

Midgley JP, Matthew AG, Greenwood CM et al 1996 Effect of reduced dietary sodium on blood pressure: a meta-analysis of randomized controlled trials. Journal of the American Medical Association 275: 1590–1597

Morimoto A, Uzu T, Fujii T et al 1997 Sodium sensitivity and cardiovascular events in patients with essential hypertension. Lancet 350: 1734–1737

Royal College of Physicians of London 1998 Clinical management of obese patients, with particular reference to the use of drugs. Royal College of Physicians, London

Willett WC, Dietz WH, Colditz GA 1999 Guidelines for healthy weight. New England Journal of Medicine 341: 427–434

Chapter 7

Briggs GC 1998 Drugs in pregnancy and lactation: a reference guide to fetal and neonatal risk, 5th edn. Williams & Wilkins, Baltimore

Brown MJ, Palmer CR, Castaigne A et al 2000 Morbidity and mortality in patients randomised to double-blind treatment with a long-acting calcium-channel blocker or diuretic in the International Nifedipine GITS study: Intervention as a Goal in Hypertension Treatment (INSIGHT). Lancet 356: 366–372

Dickerson JEC, Hingorani AD, Palmer CR et al 1999 Optimization of antihypertensive treatment by crossover rotation of four major classes. Lancet 353: 2008–2013

Estacio RO, Jeffers BW, Hiatt WR et al 1998 The effect of nisoldipine as compared with enalapril on cardiovascular outcomes in patients with non-insulin-dependent diabetes and hypertension. New England Journal of Medicine 338: 645–652

Freemantle N, Cleland J, Young P et al 1999 Beta blockade after myocardial infarction: systematic review and meta regression analysis. British Medical Journal 318: 1730–1737

Furberg CD, Psaty BM, Meyer JV 1995 Nifedipine. Dose-related increase in mortality in patients with coronary heart disease. Circulation 92: 1326–1331

Glorioso N, Troffa C, Filigheddu F et al 2000 Effect of the HMG-CoA reductase inhibitors on blood pressure in patients with essential hypertension and primary hypercholesterolemia. Hypertension 34: 1281–1286

Grimm RH Jr, Grandits GA, Prineas RJ et al 1997 Long-term effects on sexual function of five antihypertensive drugs and nutritional hygienic treatment in hypertensive men and women. Treatment of Mild Hypertension Study (TOMHS). Hypertension 29: 8–14

Hansson L, Lindholm LH, Ekbom T et al 1999a Randomised trial of old and new antihypertensive drugs in elderly patients: cardiovascular mortality and morbidity the Swedish Trial in Old Patients with Hypertension-2 study. Lancet 354: 1751–1756

Hansson L, Lindholm LH, Niskanen L et al 1999b Effect of angiotensin-converting-enzyme inhibition compared with conventional therapy on cardiovascular morbidity and mortality in hypertension: the Captopril Prevention Project (CAPPP) randomised trial. Lancet 353: 611–616

Hansson L, Hedner T, Lund-Johansen P et al 2000 Randomised trial of effects of calcium antagonists compared with diuretics and beta-blockers on cardiovascular morbidity and mortality in hypertension: the Nordic Diltiazem (NORDIL) study. Lancet 356: 359–365

Howe PR 1997 Dietary fats and hypertension. Focus on fish oil. Annals of the New York Academy of Sciences 827: 339–352

Kasiske BL, Ma JZ, Kalil RS et al 1995 Effects of antihypertensive therapy on serum lipids. Annals of Internal Medicine 122: 133–141

Kitiyakara C, Wilcox CS 1998 Antioxidants for hypertension. Current Opinion in Nephrology and Hypertension 7: 531–538

Knapp HR, FitzGerald GA 1989 The antihypertensive effects of fish oil. A controlled study of polyunsaturated fatty acid supplements in essential hypertension. New England Journal of Medicine 320: 1037–1043

Lewis EJ, Hunsicker LG, Clarke WR et al 2001 Renoprotective effect of the angiotensin-receptor antagonist irbesartan in patients with nephropathy due to type 2 diabetes. New England Journal of Medicine 345: 851–860

Messerli FH 2000 Implications of discontinuation of doxazosin arm of ALLHAT. Antihypertensive and Lipid-Lowering Treatment to Prevent Heart Attack Trial. Lancet 355: 863–864

Messerli FH, Grossman E, Goldbourt U 1998 Are beta-blockers efficacious as first-line therapy for hypertension in the elderly? A systematic review. Journal of the American Medical Association 279: 1903–1907

MRC Working Party 1992 Medical Research Council trial of treatment of hypertension in older adults: principal results. British Medical Journal 304: 405–412

Neal B, MacMahon S, Chapman N 2000 Effects of ACE inhibitors, calcium antagonists, and other blood-pressure-lowering drugs: results of prospectively designed overviews of randomised trials. Blood Pressure Lowering Treatment Trialists' Collaboration. Lancet 356: 1955–1964

Packer M, O'Connor CM, Ghali JK et al 1996 Effect of amlodipine on morbidity and mortality in severe chronic heart failure. Prospective Randomized Amlodipine Survival Evaluation Study Group. New England Journal of Medicine 335: 1107–1114

Parving HH, Lehnert H, Brochner-Mortensen J et al 2001 The effect of irbesartan on the development of diabetic nephropathy in patients with type 2 diabetes. New England Journal of Medicine 345: 870–878

Patten SB 1990 Propranolol and depression: evidence from the antihypertensive trials. Canadian Journal of Psychiatry 35: 257–259

Staessen JA, Wang JG, Thijs L 2001
Cardiovascular protection and blood
pressure reduction: a meta-analysis.
Lancet 358: 1305–1315

Stokes GS, Ryan M 1997 Can extended-
release isosorbide mononitrate be used as
an adjunctive therapy for systolic
hypertension? An open study employing
pulse wave analysis to determine effects of
antihypertensive therapy. American
Journal of Geriatric Cardiology 6: 11–19

Tatti P, Pahor M, Byington RP et al 1998
Outcome results of the Fosinopril Versus
Amlodipine Cardiovascular Events
Randomized Trial (FACET) in patients
with hypertension and NIDDM. Diabetes
Care 21: 597–603

UK Prospective Diabetes Study (UKPDS)
Group 1998 Tight blood pressure control
and risk of macrovascular and
microvascular complications in type II
diabetes: UKPDS 38. British Medical
Journal 317: 703–712

Yusuf S, Sleight P, Pogue J et al 2000 Effects
of an angiotensin-converting-enzyme
inhibitor, ramipril, on cardiovascular
events in high-risk patients. The Heart
Outcomes Prevention Evaluation Study
Investigators. New England Journal of
Medicine 342: 145–153

Chapter 8

Fletcher AE, Franks PJ, Bulpitt CJ 1988 The
effect of withdrawing antihypertensive
therapy: a review. Journal of Hypertension
6: 431–436

Hansson L, Zanchetti A, Carruthers SG et al
1998 Effects of intensive blood-pressure
lowering and low-dose aspirin in patients
with hypertension: principal results of the
Hypertension Optimal Treatment (HOT)
randomised trial. HOT Study Group.
Lancet 351: 1755–1762

Haynes RB, Sackett DL, Gibson ES 1976
Improvement of medication compliance
in uncontrolled hypertension. Lancet
1: 1265–1268

Mallion JM, Baguet JP, Siche JP 1998
Compliance, electronic monitoring and
antihypertensive drugs. Journal of
Hypertension 16: S75–S79

Medical Research Council's General Practice
Research Framework 1998 Thrombosis
prevention trial: randomised trial of low-
intensity oral anticoagulation with
warfarin and low-dose aspirin in the
primary prevention of ischaemic heart
disease in men at increased risk. Lancet
351: 233–241

Merlo J, Ranstam J, Liedholm H et al 1996
Incidence of myocardial infarction in
elderly men being treated with
antihypertensive drugs: population based
cohort study. British Medical Journal
313: 457–461

Ramsay L, Williams B, Johnston G et al 1999
Guidelines for management of
hypertension: report of the third working
party of the British Hypertension Society.
Journal of Human Hypertension
13: 569–592

Stephenson J 1999 Noncompliance may
cause half of antihypertensive drug
'failures'. Journal of the American Medical
Association 282: 313–314

Yusuf S, Sleight P, Pogue J 2000 Effects of
an angiotensin-converting-enzyme
inhibitor, ramipril, on cardiovascular
events in high-risk patients. The Heart
Outcomes Prevention Evaluation Study
Investigators. New England Journal of
Medicine 342: 145–153

Chapter 9

Bonelli FS, McKusick MA, Textor SC et al
1995 Renal artery angioplasty: technical
results and clinical outcome in 320 patients.
Mayo Clinic Proceedings 70: 1041–1052

Brown MJ, Allison DJ, Jenner DA et al 1981
Increased sensitivity and accuracy of
phaeochromocytoma diagnosis achieved
by use of plasma-adrenaline estimations
and a pentolinium-suppression test.
Lancet 1: 174–177

Geller DS, Farhi A, Pinkerton N et al 2000 Activating mineralocorticoid receptor mutation in hypertension exacerbated by pregnancy. Science 289: 119–123

Irony I, Kater CE, Biglieri EG et al 1990 Correctable subsets of primary aldosteronism. Primary adrenal hyperplasia and renin responsive adenoma. American Journal of Hypertension 3: 576–582

Jacquot C, Idatte JM, Bedrossian J et al 1978 Long-term blood pressure changes in renal homotransplantation. Archives of Internal Medicine 138: 233–236

Liddle GW, Bledsoe T, Coppage WS 1966 A familiar renal disorder simulating primary aldosteronism but with negligible aldosterone secretion. Transactions of the Association of Physicians 76: 199–213

Stewart PM, Corrie JE, Shackleton CH et al 1988 Syndrome of apparent mineralocorticoid excess. A defect in the cortisol–cortisone shuttle. Journal of Clinical Investigation 82: 340–349

Sutherland DJ, Ruse JL, Laidlaw JC 1966 Hypertension, increased aldosterone secretion and low plasma renin activity relieved by dexamethasone. Canadian Medical Association Journal 95: 1109–1119

van Jaarsveld BC, Krijnen P, Pieterman H et al 2000 The effect of balloon angioplasty on hypertension in atherosclerotic renal-artery stenosis. Dutch Renal Artery Stenosis Intervention Cooperative Study Group. New England Journal of Medicine 342: 1007–1014

Chapter 10

Agardh CD, Garcia-Puig J, Charbonnel B et al 1996 Greater reduction of urinary albumin excretion in hypertensive type II diabetic patients with incipient nephropathy by lisinopril than by nifedipine. Journal of Human Hypertension 10: 185–192

Cooper ME 1998 Pathogenesis, prevention, and treatment of diabetic nephropathy. Lancet 352: 213–219

Haffner S, Lehto S, Ronnemaa T et al 1998 Mortality from coronary heart disease in subjects with type 2 diabetes and in non-diabetic subjects with and without prior myocardial infarction. New England Journal of Medicine 339: 229–234

Hypertension in Diabetes Study (HDS) 1993 I. Prevalence of hypertension in newly presenting type 2 diabetic patients and the association with risk factors for cardiovascular and diabetic complications. Journal of Hypertension 11: 309–317

Ramsay LE, Williams B, Johnston GD et al 1999 Guidelines for management of hypertension: report of the Third Working Party of the British Hypertension Society. Journal of Human Hypertension; 13: 569–592

UK Prospective Diabetes Study (UKPDS) Group 1998a Tight blood pressure control and risk of macrovascular and microvascular complications in type II diabetes: UKPDS 38. British Medical Journal 317: 703–712

UK Prospective Diabetes Study (UKPDS) Group 1998b Intensive blood-glucose control with sulphonylureas or insulin compared with conventional treatment and risk of complications in patients with type II diabetes: UKPDS 33. Lancet 352: 837–853

Chapter 11

Burt VL, Whelton P, Roccella EJ et al 1995 Prevalence of hypertension in the US adult population. Results from the Third National Health and Nutrition Examination Survey, 1988–1991. Hypertension 25: 305–313

Dahlof B, Lindholm LH, Hansson L et al 1991 Morbidity and mortality in the Swedish Trial in Old Patients with Hypertension (STOP-Hypertension). Lancet 338: 1281–1285

Dickerson JEC, Brown MJ 1995 Influence of age on general practitioners' definition and treatment of hypertension. British Medical Journal 310: 574

Franklin SS, Gustin IVW, Wong ND et al 1997 Hemodynamic patterns of age-related changes in blood pressure: The Framingham Heart Study. Circulation 96: 308–315

Franklin SS, Jacobs MJ, Wong ND et al 2001 Predominance of isolated systolic hypertension among middle-aged and elderly US hypertensives: analysis based on national health and nutrition examination survey (NHANES) III. Hypertension 37: 869–874

Gueyffier F, Bulpitt C, Boissel JP et al 1999 Antihypertensive drugs in very old people: a subgroup meta-analysis of randomised controlled trials. INDANA Group. Lancet 353: 793–796

Hansson L, Lindholm LH, Ekbom T et al 1999 Randomised trial of old and new antihypertensive drugs in elderly patients: cardiovascular mortality and morbidity the Swedish Trial in Old Patients with Hypertension-2 study. Lancet 354: 1751–1756

Jackson R 1998 Which elderly patients should be considered for anti-hypertensive treatment? An evidence-based approach. Journal of Human Hypertension 12: 607–613

Messerli FH, Grossman E, Goldbourt U 1998 Are beta-blockers efficacious as first-line therapy for hypertension in the elderly? A systematic review. Journal of the American Medical Association 279: 1903–1907

Mulrow C, Lau J, Cornell J et al 2000 Pharmacotherapy for hypertension in the elderly (Cochrane Review). The Cochrane Library. Update Software, Oxford

Nielsen WB, Vestbo J, Jensen GB 1995 Isolated systolic hypertension as a major risk factor for stroke and myocardial infarction and an unexploited source of cardiovascular prevention: a prospective population-based study. Journal of Human Hypertension 9: 175–180

O'Donnell CJ, Ridker PM et al 1997 Hypertension and borderline isolated systolic hypertension increase risks of cardiovascular disease and mortality in male physicians. Circulation 95: 1132–1137

Primatesta P, Brookes M, Poulter NR 2001 Improved hypertension management and control: results from the health survey for England 1998. Hypertension 38: 827–832

Sagie A, Larson MG, Levy D 1993 The natural history of borderline systolic hypertension. New England Journal of Medicine 329: 1912–17

Staessen JA, Fagard R, Thijs L et al 1997 Randomised double-blind comparison of placebo and active treatment for older patients with isolated systolic hypertension. The Systolic Hypertension in Europe (Syst-Eur) Trial Investigators. Lancet 350: 757–764

van Popele NM, Bos WJ, de Beer NA et al 2000 Arterial stiffness as underlying mechanism of disagreement between an oscillometric blood pressure monitor and a sphygmomanometer. Hypertension 36: 484–488

Wilking SV, Belanger A, Kannel WB et al 1988 Determinants of isolated systolic hypertension. Journal of the American Medical Association 260: 3451–3455

Chapter 12

Bernheim J 1997 Hypertension in pregnancy. Nephron 76: 254–263

Bigrigg A, Evans M, Gbolade B et al 1999 Depo provera. Position paper on clinical use, effectiveness and side effects. British Journal of Family Planning 25: 69–76

Brown MA, Whitworth JA 1999 Management of hypertension in pregnancy. Clinical and Experimental Hypertension 21: 907–916

Chasan-Taber L, Willett WC, Manson JE et al 1996 Prospective study of oral contraceptives and hypertension among women in the United States. Circulation 94: 483–489

Dekker G, Sibai B. Primary, secondary, and tertiary prevention of pre-eclampsia. Lancet 2001: 357: 209–215

Feldman DM 2001 Blood pressure monitoring during pregnancy. Blood Pressure Monitoring 6: 1–7

Hulley S, Grady D, Bush T et al 1998 Randomized trial of estrogen plus progestin for secondary prevention of coronary heart disease in postmenopausal women. Heart and Estrogen/progestin Replacement Study (HERS) Research Group. Journal of the American Medical Association 280: 605–613

Livingston JC, Sibai BM 2001 Chronic hypertension in pregnancy. Obstetrics and Gynecology Clinics of North America; 28: 447–463

Roberts JM, Cooper DW 2001 Pathogenesis and genetics of pre-eclampsia. Lancet 357: 53–56

Task Force on Oral Contraceptives 1989 WHO Special Programme of Research, Development and Research Training in Human Reproduction. WHO multicentre trial of the vasopressor effects of combined oral contraceptives: 1. Comparisons with IUD. Contraception 40: 129–145

Writing Group for the PEPI Trial 1995 Effects of estrogen or estrogen/progestin regimens on heart disease risk factors in postmenopausal women. The Postmenopausal Estrogen/Progestin Interventions (PEPI) Trial. Journal of the American Medical Association 273: 199–208

Chapter 13

de Swiet M, Dillon MJ, Littler W et al 1989 Measurement of blood pressure in children. British Medical Journal 299: 497

Flynn JT 2001 Evaluation and management of hypertension in childhood. Progress in Pediatric Cardiology 12: 177–188

Lauer RM, Clarke WR 1989 Childhood risk factors for high adult blood pressure: the Muscatine Study. Pediatrics 84: 633–641

O'Rourke MF, Vlachopoulos C, Graham RM 2000 Spurious systolic hypertension in youth. Vascular Medicine 5: 141–145

Temple ME, Nahata MC 2000 Treatment of pediatric hypertension. Pharmacotherapy 20: 140–150

FURTHER READING

Chapter 1

Pickering TG, Coats A, Mallion JM 1999 Blood Pressure Monitoring. Task force V: White coat hypertension. Blood Pressure Monitoring 4:333–341

Strandberg TE, Salomaa V 2000 White coat effect, blood pressure and mortality in men: prospective cohort study. European Heart Journal 21:1647–1648

Vaughan CJ, Delanty D 2000 Hypertensive emergencies. Lancet 356:411–417

Chapter 3

Beutler JJ, Koomans HA 1997 Malignant hypertension: still a challenge. Nephrology Dialysis Transplantation 12:2019–2023

Chapter 8

Urquhart J 1999 The impact of drug compliance on drug development. Transplantation Proceedings 31(Suppl 4A):39S

Urquhart J, De Klerk E 1998 Contending paradigms for the interpretation of data on patient compliance with therapeutic drug regimens. Statistics in Medicine 17:251–267

Chapter 12

Duley L, Henderson-Smart DJ 2000 Drugs for rapid treatment of very high blood pressure during pregnancy. Cochrane Database of Systematic Reviews (2):CD001449

Garovic VD 2000 Hypertension in pregnancy: diagnosis and treatment. Mayo Clinic Proceedings 75:1071–1076

LIST OF PATIENT QUESTIONS

INDEX

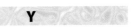